Psychological War Trauma and Society

This book explores the psychological trauma affecting soldiers and civilians who have encountered the violence of war or terrorism, arguing that the enigmas surrounding war trauma are rooted in culture, collective memory and social norms. Focusing primarily on a large-scale sociological study in Israel, chapters detail the ideological, political, historical and economic factors that shape the multifaceted connection between individual and collective trauma, probing the exterior layers of Israeli society and exposing the complex relationship between society and emotionally scarred individuals everywhere.

Divided into three main parts, particular attention is paid to the treatment of soldiers and civilians, and the tension between the medical and societal approaches to PTSD, shedding light on the intricate relationships between war trauma and society worldwide. Part I looks at traumatized soldiers and the changing attitudes towards CSR and PTSD; Part II explores civilian trauma and shock, including the first published research on the implications of war trauma in Israeli Arab society; and Part III analyses the deficiencies and contradictions in current international definitions and discourses of trauma, and the profound consequences of war trauma in society as a whole.

Psychological War Trauma and Society will be of key value for academics and postgraduate students in the fields of psychology, sociology, history, Jewish studies, military studies, social work, terrorism studies and political science, as well as professionals who work with traumatised individuals, either directly or indirectly, including psychologists, psychotherapists and social workers. The Hebrew edition of the book was the winner of the 2012 AIS (Association for Israel Studies) Shapiro Award for Best Book in Israel Studies.

Irit Keynan is Senior Lecturer and Head of the Graduate Program for Education, Society and Culture, College for Academic Studies, Or Yehuda, Israel. She is also the author of two award winning books.

Explorations in Social Psychology Series

Books in this series:

Rhetoric, Ideology and Social Psychology
Essays in honour of Michael Billig
Edited by Charles Antaki and Susan Condor

Terrorism, Trauma & Psychology
A multilevel victim perspective of the Bali bombings
Gwendoline Patricia Brookes, Julie Ann Pooley and Jaya Earnest

Psychological War Trauma and Society
Like a hidden wound
Irit Keynan

Psychological War Trauma and Society

Like a Hidden Wound

Irit Keynan

Routledge
Taylor & Francis Group
LONDON AND NEW YORK

First published in Hebrew as *Like a Hidden Wound: War Trauma in Israeli Society* 2012
by Am Oved

First published *Psychological War Trauma and Society: Like a hidden wound* 2015
by Routledge

2 Park Square, Milton Park, Abingdon, Oxfordshire OX14 4RN
711 Third Avenue, New York, NY 10017

Routledge is an imprint of the Taylor & Francis Group, an informa business

First issued in paperback 2017

British Library Cataloguing-in-Publication Data
A catalogue record for this book is available from the British Library

Library of Congress Cataloging-in-Publication Data
Keynan, Irit, author.
[Ke-'ilu hi petsa' nistar. English]
Psychological war trauma and society : like a hidden wound / Irit Keynan.
p. ; cm.
Includes bibliographical references and index.
First published in Hebrew as Like a hidden wound : war trauma in Israeli society, 2012 by Am Oved.
I. Title.
[DNLM: 1. Stress Disorders, Post-Traumatic—psychology—Israel.
2. Combat Disorders—psychology—Israel. 3. Middle East—Israel.
4. Military Personnel—Israel. 5. Social Alienation—Israel.
6. Terrorism—psychology—Israel. WM 172.5]
RC552.P67
616.85'2120095694—dc23
2014038934

ISBN: 978-1-138-84643-2 (hbk)
ISBN: 978-0-8153-5615-8 (pbk)

Typeset in Baskerville
by Apex CoVantage, LLC

This book is based on the Hebrew version of "Like a hidden wound – war trauma and Israeli society", which was researched and published with support of NATAL, Israeli Center for Trauma Victims.

To my beloved granddaughters, Dannie and Maya, may you not know war.

Contents

Acknowledgments

This book is based on the Hebrew version of my book *Like a Hidden Wound—War Trauma and Israeli Society*, which was researched and published with support of NATAL, Israel's Trauma Center for Victims of Terror and War. This book was made possible thanks to a great many people and organizations, and I am thankful to all of them. I am grateful to NATAL and in particular its founding chair, Judith Yovel Recanati, for providing the initial impetus for this study and for her moral and financial support during the research and the publication stages of the Hebrew version. My appreciation goes also to other members of NATAL: Orly Gal, Professor Avi Bleich, Dr. Itamar Barnea, Sa'ar Uziely, Sigal Haimov Dor, and Bina Levin.

The early stages of the writing were spent at New York University's Taub Center for Israel Studies. I would like to take this opportunity to express my thanks to the Center's director, Professor Ron Zweig, for the wonderful year I spent there, untroubled by everyday cares and free to focus on my writing. I also would like to thank Professor Zweig and New York University's Taub Center for Israel Studies for financial assistance and moral support concerning the English translation and expansions.

Special thanks go to Professor David Chen, for reading and offering illuminating comments on the manuscript, and for discussions that helped me to resolve some complex issues and questions. I am grateful to Professor Avraham (Rami) Friedman for the long and enlightening conversations on the complexities of interactions between victims of war trauma and the establishment, and for offering valuable comments on the Hebrew version of the manuscript.

Thanks are due also to several organizations and individuals working on war trauma who generously provided me with data and information: Miri Shalit, director of Rehabilitation Services for the Dan [Tel Aviv] District in the Defense Ministry's Rehabilitation Division; Haim Bar, chair of the Israel Defense Forces (IDF) Disabled Veterans Organization; Haim Ronen, the organization's director-general; Knesset member Israel Hasson; and Zvika Shahak, chair of the Terror Victims Association. To many severely injured war veterans I extend my gratitude for fascinating discussions that introduced me to the inner world of soldiers suffering from post-traumatic stress disorder and their unending struggle to lead "normal" lives.

Erez Zverling observingly read the entire Hebrew text, a task greatly appreciated. I am grateful to my friends Irit Tamir, for her comments on the manuscript and for encouraging me to write the epilogue, and Iris Arkin, for her unconditional support throughout the many days I was consumed by this book. I am also indebted to Dr. Yali Hashash, who helped me as a research assistant in the early stages of my research leading to writing this book, and to Tzameret Hershko for a great job of data collection.

I am grateful to Renee Hochman for editing the translation of this book, going through it meticulously and efficiently and bringing the spirit of the Hebrew version into English. Her outstanding comments also led me to a sharper interpretation of my own arguments. I am greatly indebted to her for all of these and for the enjoyable experience of working with her.

It is a pleasure to thank all of the staff at Routledge for the fascinating process of preparing the book for publication.

Above all I wish to thank those nearest and dearest to me: my children, Lilach and Nimrod, and my partner, Itzik. My beloved children allowed me to see the issue of war trauma through the eyes of young post-army Israelis, and showered me with unconditional love and support throughout the writing process. I thank Lilach for helping me see how painful Israeli reality is and how difficult it is to distance oneself from it, and Nimrod for the engrossing conversations we shared about the human soul and its ability to detach and repress its anxieties.

Itzik, whose love and support are an ever-present light in my life, gave me the much needed tranquility during the emotionally intense writing process. I also thank him for being a wise and careful critic, the first to read and comment on every page of the book; and for his wonderful ability to give me the space I need for creative work, and at the same time be available whenever I need his support.

Introduction to the Non-Israeli Reader

As I was working on the final draft of this book, an article in *Time* magazine attracted my attention (Thompson 2014). It reported that while approximately 125,000 or 5% of the 2.5 million American troops in Afghanistan and Iraq have been diagnosed with PTSD, a new congressional sponsored study found that the real figure was even higher: 8%, or 200,000 veterans. Two months earlier, Australian Defense Forces estimated a comparable percentage of PTSD wounded among their veterans who served in Iraq and Afghanistan (Brown 2014). The proportion of PTSD sufferers among combatants in Israel is also similar. These figures from diverse wars and countries underscore the universal scope of war trauma in present-day battles fought by Western countries.

Unfortunately, we cannot expect to see a drop in the number of war victims, including war trauma victims, in the near future. Many new armed conflicts have flared up in different parts of the world, while other long-standing conflicts have persisted without resolution. Too many to note individually, I will mention only three salient war situations: a new conflict has emerged between Russia and the Ukraine; in Syria thousands of people are killed every week in clashes between the government and insurgents; and in Iraq, the Islamic State (ISIS) militants leave terror and horror in their wake wherever they go, prompting renewed intervention by the US and probably other countries. Despite the huge numbers of psychological war-trauma casualties in these wars, the hidden wounds are those less told, and even today, remain stigmatized; they represent the war toll that societies find difficult to acknowledge, although all armies know that many of their combatants will suffer war trauma and forever change.

As I am writing this introduction, a war is raging between Israel and the Hamas[1] in Gaza, reminding me that the Hebrew version of the book was published during another war in Gaza, in 2012. Although I live about 40 miles from Israel's southern border, I was, then and now, frequently shaken by the sounds of sirens going off, rushing me to the shelter for protection against rocket fire (4,000 rockets were launched at Israel, including Tel Aviv, over the last two months). Thanks to the Iron Dome,[2] these rockets failed to cause significant damage in the center of Israel, but citizens in proximity to the border suffered enormously both from rockets (the Iron Dome cannot intercept rockets fired from a close distance) and from attempts of Hamas militants to strike civilian towns through underground tunnels.

This situation naturally affected the Israeli civilian population, and as far as figures are available, Israel's health care services have treated hundreds of civilians suffering from acute stress in this recent conflict. How many have decided not to come forward, and how many will develop PTSD, it is still early to know. The Israeli population undeniably has lived under almost constant threat for decades. Since Israel's founding in 1948, over 3,000 hostile acts were inflicted against civilians in addition to three full-scale wars and several moderate-scale wars. Palestinian civilians also suffer tremendously, both physical destruction and psychological trauma. At the time of writing this introduction, estimates of civilian Palestinian casualties in Gaza stand at over 1,000 dead, 10,000 wounded, and tens of thousands displaced from their homes. It is too early to predict the psychological damage of the civilians in Gaza.

Unfortunately, in the last two decades, terror continues to extend its reach, and many Western countries that have not known wars or security threats for decades have come under this cloud of violence. This book, exploring the relations between psychological war trauma and society, is based mainly on the experience of Israel, and to a lesser extent on that of the US, but the growing prevalence of terror and the universality of many of the features and implications of psychological war trauma make this book relevant to readers everywhere.

The intricate relationship between society and war trauma is influenced by historical contingencies, social forces, and what anthropologist Allan Young calls "epistemic culture" (Duclos 2013). Thus, while each society has its own specific ways of understanding war trauma, Western societies share many common patterns for coping with it. This makes the Israeli experience instructive and helpful, as it sheds light on other societies as well, highlighting the common aspects of war trauma alongside those that are unique to Israeli circumstances. To enhance the book's appeal for the international reader, this translation from the Hebrew version (Keynan 2012) has been expanded to include practical information about war trauma in other countries, and wherever appropriate, the universality of phenomena observed in Israel was underscored.

The war around me, which feels like a suitably macabre décor for writing a book on trauma, took on a special personal twist one day, when one of my students told me that his 23-year-old son came back from the war acting erratically. From the description of his behavior I understood that he suffered a combat stress reaction. I tried to help by referring him to the army unit that to my best knowledge offers the finest treatment available, as my heart went out to the young man and his family, foreseeing the ordeals they will be facing for many years to come. I then recalled a long, moving conversation I had with an American veteran whom I had met in New York at 2009, and who later became a friend. On September 11, he was among those who were sent to bring out the firefighters and members of other rescue forces who were killed or injured in the World Trade Center. He later served in Iraq for eight months, and was among those who supposedly came back safe and sound. A year later, PTSD erupted without warning. He lost his job, and lost himself, and ended up homeless for many months, struggling to obtain help from the VA. "When you come back from Iraq," he said, "there is no one you can talk to. The world is so different, you feel like an alien. Friends and family prefer not to hear about the war, and you feel like the loneliest person on earth" (CD/IK 2009).

A few days later, I received another call; it was one of my students, who wanted to share her distress with me. Whenever the sirens go off, she said, she could not control her physiological reactions—sweating, shivering, sometimes fainting. She said she knew it was irrational, but her body was unwilling to comply with this understanding. She said she had not left her house for weeks, for fear of a siren going off, catching her far from a shelter. Talking with her for a long time, explaining the symptoms of acute stress and urging her to see a therapist, I thought about all the individuals, wherever they are, who do not have someone to talk to about their experiences with PTSD, and carry this unbearable wound inside them, sometimes hidden from sight for years and years.

There are countless people around us who feel this way. This book is dedicated to them, with the hope that societies will finally start thinking about this unspoken toll of war, and work to find another path into a better, more peaceful future.

Irit Keynan, Tel Aviv, August 2014

Notes

1. An Islamic terrorist movement, based in the Gaza strip between Egypt and Israel.
2. Mobile air defense system developed by Israeli Rafael Advanced Defense Systems, to intercept and destroy short-range rockets and artillery shells fired from distances of 4 kilometers (2.5 miles) to 70 kilometers (43 miles) away and whose trajectory would take them to a populated area.

References

Brown, R. 2014 'Australian Defence Force Veterans Detail Growing Scourge of Post-Traumatic Stress Disorder', *ABC News (Australian Broadcasting Corporation)*, 23 April. Available from www.abc.net.au/news/2014-04-23/rising-ptsd-compensation-figures-in-adf-only-the-start/5404778 [10 August 2014].

CD/IK confidential interview, 2009.

Duclos, V. 2013 'When Anthropology Meets Science: an Interview with Allan Young'. Available from http://somatosphere.net/2013/10/when-anthropology-meets-science-an-interview-with-allan-young.html [8 August 2014].

Keynan, I. 2012, *Like a Hidden Wound: War Trauma in Israeli Society*. Am Oved, Tel Aviv.

Thompson, M. 2014, 'The PTSD Epidemic: Many Suffering, Few Solutions', *Time*, 20 June. Available from http://time.com/2904783/ptsd-iraq-va [24 July 2014].

Introduction

War Trauma, Myth, and Longing in Israeli Society

For a century the world ignored the existence of post-traumatic stress disorder (PTSD). A full hundred years passed between the initial discoveries made by Freud, Breuer, and Janet regarding psychological trauma and its acceptance as a legitimate medical syndrome. During that century, those afflicted with posttraumatic stress were abandoned to their misery and often accused of faking their symptoms, shirking their duties, and trying to wangle financial compensation. This egregiously delayed acceptance of PTSD owed not to a lack of knowledge or even the absence of scientific study of the subject. Instead, it was the result of a broad failure on the part of psychologists and policymakers to recognize that psychological trauma is not rooted in personality disorder but is, rather, an injury induced by external forces, particularly by violent acts perpetrated by human beings. Recognition of war trauma, says Judith Lewis Herman, in most cases, requires an individual to take a moral stance regarding the events in question. Yet a great temptation exists to ignore evil—not to see it, not to hear it, not to talk about it (Herman 1997). Denial of the existence of PTSD stemmed also from ideological and economic factors and the competing perceptions and ego-conflicts between and within relevant professions. Physicians found it hard to abandon old paradigms, insurance companies feared the ensuing claims should the syndrome be recognized, military leaders saw it as a threat to the myth of the fearless warrior, while for pacifists, PTSD signaled only inappropriate behavior by soldiers during war. All of this placed the issue of psychological trauma at the center of intense and ideologically charged disputes, preventing the assimilation of scientific findings on the topic and leading to a kind of "episodic amnesia" (Herman 1997, p. 7), a forgetting of existing knowledge and a consequent need to rediscover it, again and again. While, for example, US Army chief of psychiatry Thomas W. Salmon had formulated a set of principles for the treatment of traumatized soldiers during World War I (WWI), these had been abandoned by the Second World War (WWII), and the American military entered the war without any personnel trained to deal with trauma.

Psychological trauma is precipitated by events of various kinds, both manmade—war, sexual violence, and other crimes—and accidents or natural disasters. This book focuses on trauma caused by violence in a context of national conflict—namely, war and terrorism. The book looks mostly at Israel, but it brings incisive insights for all nations facing these harmful situations. War leaves emotional scars on all who take part: defeated or victor, soldier or civilian. Recovery involves overcoming painful memories, coping with loss and with questions of meaning, and reassembling the puzzle of one's life, making the pre- and postwar pieces fit together. Most of those exposed to war manage, through a gradual process, to put the horror behind them. However, by current estimates, about 15% are unable to heed the call of daily life after war or terror experiences. Though to all appearances they have returned safe and sound and without injury, they find no balm for their wounds. Their pain is invisible, and they are often left with feelings of solitude, the din of carnage refusing to fade. These are the bloodless victims, those psychologically traumatized by war.[1]

Psychological trauma causes significant functional disability and profound suffering and does not readily respond to psychotherapy or drug therapy. It appears in the wake of exposure to violence or threat to one's life or physical integrity. Sometimes witnessing injury or the threat of injury to another can also cause a traumatic reaction, as can learning of the violent, sudden death of a loved one. Trauma can manifest itself in different ways from the time of the triggering event over the course of the victim's life.[2]

Psychological trauma experienced by soldiers during or immediately after combat is called *combat stress reaction* (CSR). This term, which replaced numerous predecessors, denotes an acute stress reaction leading to behavioral change and to impaired personal and military functional capacity, to the point of inability to continue fighting (Bleich & Melamed 2007).[3] CSR is not the "regular" kind of distress induced by the hardships of war. It is an injury, however, to the psyche rather than the body. It can accompany physical injury or it can appear separately, a wound that cannot be bandaged. Its typical symptoms are shock, emotional detachment, difficulty responding to one's environment, and dysfunction that make a soldier unable to continue fighting even when his life is in immediate danger.[4] Soldiers may also be traumatized by their involvement in actions that bring serious physical or emotional injury to others, especially civilians, a trauma associated with a sense of weighty moral conflict.[5]

In most cases, a traumatic reaction subsides on its own, and the sufferer recovers relatively quickly. However, reactions sometimes persist for an extended period following the traumatic event, compromising the victim's ability to function in later life. In some instances, the onset of symptoms is delayed and the syndrome manifests only after life has ostensibly returned to normal.[6]

The definition of a psychologically traumatic event and the symptoms associated with psychological trauma have changed and expanded over the years, as a growing body of research has led to a more nuanced understanding of the syndrome.[7] In contrast to earlier conceptions, today's prevailing definition recognizes that one may suffer psychological trauma not only from an acute threat to one's life but also from witnessing such a threat to the life of another. For example, soldiers who, in battle, are present at scenes of severe injury, death, or atrocity can become traumatized even if their own lives are not immediately threatened, as can civilians who witness such scenes, or rescue workers involved in evacuating the wounded and the dead. According to the accepted definition of the international psychiatric establishment, sufferers of PTSD experience four types of symptoms: **Intrusion or reexperiencing**—the persistent and uncontrollable reexperiencing of the traumatic event, whether in dreams or in the form of intrusive thoughts or flashbacks; **avoidance**—an emotional numbing, repression, or sense of detachment, which serves to alleviate the distress caused by the uncontrolled recollection of distressing memories, thoughts, feelings, or external reminders of the trigger event; and **hyperarousal**—excessive sweating, nervousness, irritability, tension, difficulty sleeping, and problems concentrating, all marked by aggressive, reckless, or self-destructive behavior. *DSM-5* (American Psychiatric Association 2013) added to the previous editions a fourth cluster of **negative cognitions and mood**, which represent myriad feelings, from a persistent and distorted sense of blame of self or others to estrangement from others or markedly diminished interest in activities.[8] These symptoms manifest in the daily lives of victims in a complex pattern and in a variety of emotional reactions: they feel constant anxiety accompanied by physiological signs of fear and defensiveness; they are subject to outbursts of anger; they become withdrawn, lose interest in the things they had previously enjoyed, avoid social interaction, and seal themselves off emotionally. Many fail to reintegrate into the workplace, have trouble communicating, even with their own family members, or fear to go outsides their homes.

Among the larger group of the less severely impaired, many manage to function well at work, but their familial and social relationships suffer, sometimes irreparably. Most of those who fall into this latter category do not seek treatment, and their lives become an ongoing struggle in which they strive to gain control over the traumatic experience and to expunge it from their minds. They frequently turn to drugs or alcohol to ease the pain and to dull their thoughts and memories. The trauma takes up a major portion of their emotional energy, leaving them with little to expend on other needs.

The term combat stress reaction (CSR) is used only to denote soldiers' traumatic reaction in battle. In Israel, the traumatic reaction experienced by civilians in the wake of terrorist attacks or other violent incidents is referred to as anxiety or "shock" (*harada*). This term carries a certain stigma, implying weakness and dependence on security forces. Although the context is different, civilian "shock" manifests itself in ways similar to CSR. Civilians find themselves caught up in a violent event with no advanced preparation, generally in the course of everyday activities. The arbitrariness of this violence intensifies the shock and the consequent damage to the victim's sense of security precisely because the attack takes place within normal life. However, the victims in these instances are generally evacuated quickly from the scene of the attack, and thereby distanced from the threat to their lives. Soldiers, by contrast, are usually injured in battle, where the threat to their lives is prolonged beyond the moment of injury, and the injury itself is compounded by the emotional stress brought on by their duty to fellow soldiers. They thus experience a mortifying sense of failure and guilt due to their inability to function at such a critical time.

In this book I will be dealing with soldiers and civilians traumatized by war and terrorism. Nevertheless, it should be emphasized that trauma affects not only those directly afflicted but also their loved ones, particularly parents, spouses, and children, whose suffering is often great and can ultimately constitute a form of trauma in and of itself (Solomon et al. 1992). As noted earlier, psychological trauma can also be caused by the violent death of a loved one, and thus the category of the traumatized should also include those bereaved individuals who never recover from the knock on the door informing them of the death of a loved one in war or a terror attack.

The victims of war trauma, both soldiers and civilians, many times remain outside of existing social and institutional circles of support. In part, this owes to the nature of the syndrome, which alters the victim's consciousness and impairs his ability to maintain interpersonal relationships, thereby limiting the ability to seek and obtain help. The main explanation, however, entails a broader social context. Fear and a lack of awareness engender widespread indifference and estrangement toward victims of war trauma. Beyond the impairment it induces individually, war trauma raises serious questions at the collective level: How aware are we of the price exacted by war? What is the individual's duty to his country and the country's to the individual? To what extent is a nation obligated to sympathize with individual suffering, and how is such sympathy to be balanced with the obligations for a tough and tenacious defense of the state and its citizens? Does societal recognition of trauma, whether official or unofficial, weaken or strengthen society? Does a sense of mission and of duty to the nation insulate soldiers from a fear of death? Is war-related psychological trauma indeed an impairment of the mind, in the way that the loss of a leg or arm is an impairment of the body? Or should the disorder be perceived as a weakness, a psychosomatic illness undeserving of appreciation and dangerous to the nation as a whole? Who is a hero? What is heroism? And how do all of these issues relate to the elusive and controversial term "patriotism?"

Psychologically traumatized soldiers throughout the world have often been treated with the kind of hostility today reserved for traitors and deserters. During WWI, for example, CSR victims were sometimes executed on charges of cowardice and desertion. Examples of similar attitudes, though less extreme punishments, could be found during Israel's War of Independence, when CSR sufferers were accused of shirking their duties, subjected to derogatory name-calling, and afforded no treatment of any kind. American soldiers returning from Vietnam—and into a scene of domestic political discord—often experienced a sense of estrangement and felt themselves demonized. In this context, many who needed it avoided seeking treatment from the Department of Veterans Affairs, which, for its part, proved reluctant to acknowledge widespread PTSD among returning soldiers. The two countries witnessed similar time lines in the acknowledgment and legitimization of PTSD, though Israel preceded the US by a few years. During the 1973 Yom Kippur War, the significance—if not the scope—of war trauma began to emerge in the Israeli national consciousness. In the US, the validity of PTSD was the subject of fervent debate leading up to the syndrome's inclusion in the

DSM-3, in 1980. But in both countries, official recognition by no means ended the prejudice against war trauma-injured people, which, despite progress, remains even to this day.

In Israel, over the past four decades, we have witnessed a gradual recognition and legitimation of war-related psychological trauma. Advances and regressions have characterized this tortuous process. The idea that civilians too could be afflicted with trauma gained public recognition only during the 2000s, although large-scale civilian traumatization had been observed during the First Persian Gulf War (1991). Attention to the issue of civilian trauma built upon the growing recognition of soldiers' trauma. Awareness further increased in the wake of the World Trade Center attacks in New York in 2001 and the Second Intifada in Israel (2001–2004), during which many civilians suffered shock and fright.

While I was writing the book, it became clear that Israeli attitudes and policy concerning war trauma constitute a powerful lens through which to view and analyze broader aspects of society, and I believe the same is true for other societies. Some of the issues brought into clearer focus are the intricate interaction between the state, society, and the wounded veteran and civilian population, the ways Israeli society copes with the ongoing experience of threat, the development of myths and social beliefs, and the close, complex, and somewhat contradictory relationship between individual and collective trauma. It also became clear that in Israel, as elsewhere, attitudes toward trauma are shaped not only by "neutral" medical considerations but also by ideological, historical, and economic forces. The book elucidates these processes, tracing the shifting attitudes toward trauma in relation to broader historical developments.

The book calls attention to controversial topics that have consumed the Israel Defense Forces (IDF) and Israeli society, including the way the state has treated soldiers who have returned wounded from their service. It also addresses questions, which have plagued Israeli society in recent years, about the justification for war and the sense that once-sacred norms have begun to dissolve. These include the principle of leaving no wounded behind and the state's absolute commitment to soldiers caught behind enemy lines.

The development of Israeli attitudes toward civilian shock also has broader implications. An ongoing confusion has prevailed since the founding of the state over both the role of civilians in wartime and the state's obligation to noncombatants harmed during war. Although citizens have always been expected to take part in Israel's struggle for continued existence, the state's commitment to physically wounded civilians was limited for years. Until the 1970s, the state offered care to wounded civilians only in cases of poverty. Today, when civilians wounded in war or terrorist attacks are entitled to the same compensation as wounded soldiers, the victims of terrorism and their families are still struggling for greater acknowledgment of their sacrifice. They seek to emerge from the anonymity of accidental victimhood, to be appreciated as *soldiers without uniforms*. What is at stake is the meaning of *memorialization* and *recognition* within the Israeli warrior ethos. The families of victims of terrorism wish to be part of Israel's collective narrative of a heroic and perpetual struggle for survival. Their efforts to broaden the banner of national heroism reflect the power of a shared national narrative to confer meaning on personal loss and suffering during war.

Many factors have led to the transformation of attitudes and recent legitimation of war trauma and its victims. Among them, a special and important place is occupied by the victims themselves and by their families, the more resilient of whom have organized into self-help groups and advocacy organizations. However, despite the considerable progress that has been made, debate persists and repudiation of the claims of the war-traumatized remains widespread. Even the agencies responsible for treatment and compensation have been inadequate in their response to victims' needs. The hidden wound of psychological trauma, whose symptoms resemble the stereotypes of character weakness, continues to inspire doubt—if no longer about its existence then about its severity, its causes, and the number and reliability of those afflicted. Ideological and economic determinants still complicate the debate over psychological trauma, and one still hears arguments that such trauma is merely a social invention, one dangerous to national resilience.

In Israeli society, two main reasons account for the reluctance to accept the idea of psychological trauma: existential fears for the future of the state—fears that do not necessarily reflect geopolitical reality—and a national profound need to feel just, equally perceived as existentially important for the nation. These two themes form the basis of a national ethos of heroism and resilience, which shapes Israeli society's attitude toward security issues.

Regarding the first theme, that of existential fear, the very existence of a traumatic reaction to war poses a threat to Israel's ability to defend itself in the face of ongoing hostility, the cessation of which is widely felt to be chimeric. The very idea of trauma threatens Israelis' faith in the ability of the IDF to defend the nation. It also undermines confidence that the civilian population will remain steadfast in the face of long-term security threats. Israeli existential fear—the country's dominant collective narrative—closes off the possibility of empathy toward perceived weakness, seen as a harbinger of national exhaustion.

The second theme, Israel's need to believe in its moral superiority, engenders divergent attitudes toward two distinct groups of psychologically traumatized civilians: Israelis and Palestinians. On the one hand, the large number of nonuniformed Israeli shock victims substantiates the sense of justice that Israelis feel in their war with the Palestinians, a war widely viewed in Israel as one of self-defense. This perception makes it easier to accept civilian psychological trauma as a form of war injury, despite the implicit threat to the nation's resilience. On the other hand, it becomes difficult to acknowledge the same phenomenon when it affects enemy civilians, as this would undermine the myth of being in the right.

The myth of moral superiority encourages another type of myopia as well—not toward the trauma suffered by Palestinians, but toward that suffered by Israeli soldiers serving among Palestinian civilians in the Occupied Territories. *Moral injury*, a relatively new concept in the field of trauma studies, denotes a trauma inflicted on a soldier from "taking part in, failing to prevent, bearing witness to, or learning about acts that transgress deeply held moral beliefs and expectations" (Maguen & Litz 2012, p. 1). The possibility—evident since the 1987 First Intifada—that Israeli soldiers could suffer moral injuries, that they might become traumatized through harming civilians, poses a threat to Israeli moral authority. In the eyes of critics, the very acknowledgment of the possibility of moral injury becomes conflated with an acknowledgment of human rights violations or war crimes. It is precisely this ethical confusion and elusive sense of justice that explains the vehement denial of psychological trauma triggered in soldiers involved in harming civilians. This type of wound remains unseen and ignored by most Israelis. As expressed by a young Israeli veteran, it is a "transparent trauma" (Sharon 2005).

In short, the Israeli denial of trauma has not disappeared; it has merely changed its form and direction.

It appears somewhat paradoxical that a nation such as Israel, born of collective trauma and whose public life is deeply imbued with collective suffering, should display widespread apathy, opposition, and ambivalence toward individual suffering. The contradiction, however, is illusory. In reality, the more intense the collective sense of trauma, the more likely the collective is to close ranks and the more limited its ability to exhibit empathy toward the individual.

In a country born of and into war, the immediate reason for this inability to show empathy is virtually self-evident. Israel's War of Independence heralded the culmination of the struggle to establish a Jewish state and to solve the "Jewish problem," yet it failed to bring an end to military conflicts, a problem that plagues the state to this day. The Zionist movement emerged in the late nineteenth century as a sense of impending disaster. With these fears all too catastrophically realized in the Holocaust, the consciousness of persecution and danger became seared into the Jewish national experience. The state's founders wove existential dread into the national ethos, framing a continuous narrative between the Jewish people's bloody history of persecution and a persistent threat to Jewish national life following the long-dreamed-of return to Zion.

It would not be an exaggeration to say that Israeli society is imprisoned by its sense of impending disaster. This fact is evident in the frequent reference to collective memory of persecution in Israeli public life; in Israeli attitudes toward security issues; in the suspicion with which Israelis regard those who do not fully identify with each and every facet of their country's policy; and in a lingering feeling of transience (exemplified, for example, by the common phenomenon of obtaining an additional passport "just in case") (Levy 2011).

As early as 1983, psychologist Rafael Moses warned of the danger inherent in these processes. According to Moses, Israeli collective behavior bears striking similarities to the behavioral patterns of trauma victims. As with trauma victims, who often live with the conviction that the traumatic incident will repeat itself, Israeli collective behavior threatens to stimulate self-fulfilling prophecy (Moses 1983). The chronic national preoccupation with events that have caused collective trauma breeds an obsessive repetition of relational patterns that, as Moses sees it, recreate past persecutions. This culminates in the Israeli quest for proof of persecution in the present and the perpetuation of a sense of national victimhood. At the heart of this process lies the illusory hope of allaying fear through military might.

Israel is not the only society to exhibit such effects of collective trauma on the national psyche. Studies conducted over the past decade have shown that the aftereffects of collective trauma can linger for decades, even centuries. Traumatized groups are often characterized by existential fears and a lack of faith in the possibility of change. These latter feelings, in turn, can reinforce and intensify conflicts, even to the point of obstructing possible political resolution. Traumatized groups are also easily influenced by leaders who use the memory of trauma and the fear of its repetition to draw them again and again into military conflict (Halpern & Weinstein 2004; Keynan 2009; Volkan 2009). The workings of national trauma also help explain why people conceive of war trauma principally as afflicting their own side of a given conflict. An atmosphere of existential fear and skepticism about ever mitigating the threat encourages group insularity and limits understanding of the other side's suffering. This helps explain why the Israeli public disregarded Palestinian trauma for so many years, even among Palestinian citizens of Israel. Only in recent years, particularly since the Second Lebanon War (2006), have researchers and relevant professionals begun to devote attention, however minimal, to the effects of war on Israel's Arab citizens.

Unconscious motivations have a tremendous impact on behavior. Only by increasing our awareness of these motivations might we escape the trap of unconscious behavior and self-fulfilling prophecies (Moses 1983). In this book I argue that a close correlation exists between the manner in which Israeli society deals with the effects of war on the individual psyche and the ways it copes with its traumatic collective past and questions of national life. These two phenomena are linked by unconscious motivations. The need to face these issues and rationally address how they shape our lives and our future, together with the duty to those who pay the price of war in body and spirit, constitutes the fundamental impetus for the present work.

Over the last few years the clinical aspects of war and terrorism-related psychological trauma have garnered considerable scholarly attention. Many recent books and articles have also addressed war and terrorism-related bereavement, examining the topic's personal, social, and political implications. A vast body of research, produced over the years of Israel's existence, has examined the ramifications of the Holocaust and collective memory. But on the social, cultural, and national contexts of war trauma at the individual level, only little has been written. With this book I hope to fill the gap and to lift the veil of obscurity from the topic of war-related psychological trauma.

I wrote this book from the perspective of social history, relying on the research methodologies customarily employed by scholars of that field. The overall picture was drawn on the basis of a wide variety of sources: oral and written testimonies, interviews with trauma victims and with relevant public officials, letters, proceedings of professional and political committees, laws and records of legislative deliberation, statistics and medical data, empirical data, literature, fictional and documentary films and television shows, newspaper articles, and radio programs. I also used a myriad of scholarly studies in fields touching on history, society, culture, and the human mind. The psychological aspects of the present work are based on an extensive body of research and the writings of trauma experts all over the world. This vast swath of sources enabled me to trace the development of the discourse on trauma in different segments of society, in the medical world and in the political world, and to identify the patterns of mutual effects of socio-political and scientific processes and the perception of trauma and its victims. Analyzing all the primary and secondary sources, comparing thoughts with data, and comparing my conclusions with those of other scholars allowed me to draw a comprehensive, solid picture, which, like any study, may raise different opinions within readers.

The book is divided into three parts. Part I deals with traumatized soldiers and examines changing attitudes toward CSR and PTSD in a broader context of social and security-related developments in Israel and with attention to changing attitudes toward trauma in other nations, particularly in the US. The first two chapters of this part address the particularities of CSR and the unique predicament that can ensnare soldiers sent to battle in the name of their countries; changing attitudes toward victims of CSR around the world beginning in the early twentieth century; and the factors that hampered recognition of CSR as a legitimate injury. The third chapter analyzes how Israeli perceptions of trauma and trauma victims developed between the War of Independence and the Yom Kippur War. The fourth chapter traces advancements in the understanding and treatment of CSR since the 1980s and looks at trauma victims' present relations with the army and the Ministry of Defense. The fifth chapter deals with the debates about war in Israel over the past few decades and the ramifications of these debates on the perception of trauma. Here I track the shift in the denial of trauma to the politically sensitive subject of Israel's occupation of the Palestinian territories. The concluding chapter of this part looks at new risk factors for CSR in light of social transformations driven by privatization and globalization as well as changes in the relationship between the IDF and Israeli society.

Part II, divided into five chapters, is devoted to the topic of civilian sufferers of shock. The first analyzes the changes that have slowly taken place in the state's attitude toward civilians injured in war, culminating in the recognition of the state's duty to those wounded in war and in terrorist incidents. The second chapter looks at how the concept of civilian shock entered public discourse and the development of patterns of coping with the new phenomenon. I find the First Persian Gulf War (1991) to be the moment when the concept of individual trauma became linked to that of Jewish collective trauma. This chapter also investigates Israeli patterns of collective coping with incidents of mass shock during the Second Intifada. The third chapter explores the shaping of the discourse on civilian trauma. It elucidates changes that have occurred in the relationship between the discourse and reality of civilian trauma since the Al-Aqsa Intifada. I discuss the establishment's attitude toward victims and the role played by voluntary associations in raising awareness about war trauma and aiding those affected. The fourth chapter addresses the inner contradictions in Israeli discourse on war trauma. It analyzes the bitter and painful disagreement between the bereaved families of civilian casualties and those of fallen soldiers over the status of their loved ones on scales of national sacrifice and heroism, and the internal tension between the Israeli discourse on trauma and that on national resilience.

The final chapter in part II is especially innovative, being the first published research to explore the social complexity and implications of war trauma in Israeli Arab society. This multifaceted topic is significant for reasons both methodological and social. From a scholarly perspective, one cannot consider the Israeli citizenry without including its Arab component. From a social perspective, it is crucial to emphasize that war trauma transcends national boundaries. Israel's Arab citizens are affected by trauma just as their Jewish counterparts are, and both sides are victims of the ongoing conflict. Perhaps an awareness of this will pave the way to a new approach to the conflict and a more assiduous search for a solution.

The book's third part is devoted to further exploration of major concerns that emanate from the first two parts. I argue that an inherent deficiency exists in the present conceptualization of trauma and the scope of its definition, both in Israel and internationally. The chapter analyzes two prevailing contradictory arguments about the definition of war trauma. The first claims that the definition of war trauma is overly broad and thus self-defeating; the second views the definition as excessively narrow and incapable of reflecting the range of symptoms experienced by casualties, the social aspects of trauma, or the shadow of war that lingers in the hearts of so many. I contend that the current understanding of war trauma is incomplete, as it does not fully encompass the social role played by the psychological and psychiatric clinical discourse on war trauma. In particular, I point at the potential inner contradictions in the common attempt of psychologists to avoid the social aspects of trauma, under the guise of shunning politics. The third part—and the book as a whole—concludes with a chapter examining the trajectories of trauma discourse, from individual to collective and back again. This chapter offers a comprehensive view—painful and troubling—of the way Israeli society is dominated by a traumatized ethos, evident both in national life and in the state's international relations, and which reflects the longing of a society for what it once dreamed of becoming, but lost.

Notes

1. The figure of 15% of those exposed to war is based on follow-up and research studies carried out in Israel and the US (Bleich & Solomon, 2002). War victims are men and women. For the sake of convenience I usually use the masculine form.
2. For the kinds of events that can cause PTSD and the symptoms associated with it, see American Psychiatric Association (2013).
3. Note that combat stress reaction is a specific instance of acute stress reaction. On the kinds of stress reaction experienced over time, see note 2.
4. For the full range of symptoms and developmental stages of CSR, see Bleich (1990); Bleich and Melamed (2007); and Briere (2004).

5. This kind of injury is vividly illustrated in the opening scene of the film *Lebanon* (2009).
6. CSR and shock are specific instances of the traumatic syndrome. When the syndrome appears immediately and persists for up to two days, it is called "acute stress reaction." When it persists for up to one month it is called "acute stress disorder." Sometimes onset is delayed for weeks, months, or even years. In such cases, or in instances where it persists for more than a month, it is termed post-traumatic stress disorder (PTSD). PTSD was first accorded recognition in 1980. Its clinical definition, detailing the symptoms and the kinds of events that can cause it, appeared for the first time in the *DSM-3*, the third edition of the American Psychiatric Association's *Diagnostic and Statistical Manual of Mental Disorders*, the diagnostic handbook considered authoritative by the psychiatric establishment throughout the Western world (American Psychiatric Association 1980). Every few years the definition is updated with revisions to the DSM. For the sake of convenience I will be using the terms "trauma," "post-trauma," and "PTSD" to denote the phenomenon in a general way; occasionally I will employ the terms "combat stress reaction" and "shock"—to be explained ahead—when I wish to refer to them specifically. Extensive use will be made of the term "war trauma," on which I will elaborate separately in the book's concluding part.
7. For the 1980 definition, see American Psychiatric Association (1980). For the changes over time, see American Psychiatric Association (2000, 2013).
8. For a more extensive discussion of the symptoms, see Briere (2004) and Levin et al. (2014).

References

American Psychiatric Association 1980, *Diagnostic and Statistical Manual of Mental Disorders*, 3rd edn., Washington D.C.

American Psychiatric Association 2000, *Diagnostic and Statistical Manual of Mental Disorders*, 4th edn., Washington D.C.

American Psychiatric Association 2013, *Diagnostic and Statistical Manual of Mental Disorders*, 5th edn. Available from www.dsm5.org.

Bleich, A. 1990, 'Acute Combat Stress Reaction: Pathogenic, Diagnostic and Therapeutic Aspects', *I.D.F. Medical Corps Bulletin*, vol. 32, pp. 43–45. (Hebrew)

Bleich, A., & Melamed, Y. 2007, 'Post-Traumatic Emotional Damage and Impairment following Military Service', *Journal of Medicine and Law*, vol. 37, pp. 37–44. (Hebrew)

Bleich, A., & Solomon, Z. 2002, 'Psychiatric Evaluation of Psychiatric Disability in PTSD of Military Origin' in *Mental Disability: Medical, Research Social, Legal and Rehabilitative Aspects*, eds A. Bleich & Z. Solomon, Ministry of Defense, Tel Aviv, pp. 43–71. (Hebrew)

Briere, J. 2004, *Psychological Assessment of Adult Posttraumatic States: Phenomenology, Diagnosis, and Measurement*, 2nd edn. Washington, DC: American Psychological Association.

Halpern, J., & Weinstein, H. M. 2004, 'Rehumanizing the Other: Empathy and Reconciliation', *Human Rights Quarterly*, vol. 26, no. 3, pp. 561–583.

Herman, J. L. 1997, *Trauma and Recovery*, Basic Books, New York.

Keynan, I. 2009, 'Collective Memory and Intergroup Leadership: Israel as a Case Study', in *Crossing the Divide: Intergroup Leadership in a World of Difference*, ed T. L. Pittinsky, Harvard Business Press, Boston, pp. 219–230.

Lebanon 2009, motion picture.

Levin, A. P., Kleinman, S. B., & Adler, J. S. 2014, 'DSM-5 and Posttraumatic Stress Disorder', *Journal of the American Academy of Psychiatry and the Law Online*, vol. 42, no. 2, pp. 146–158.

Levy, G. 2011, 'Fear Is Driving Israelis to Obtain Foreign Passports', *Haaretz*, 2 June.

Maguen, S., & Litz, B. 2012, 'Moral Injury in Veterans of War', *PTSD Research Quarterly*, vol. 23, no. 1, pp. 1–6.
Moses, R. 1983, 'Emotional Response to Stress in Israel: a Psychoanalytic Perspective', in *Stress in Israel*, ed S. Breznits, Van Nostrand Reinhold, New York, pp. 114–137.
Sharon, A. 2005, 'Transparent Trauma', *Breaking the Silence*. Available from www.shovrimshtika.org/article.asp?id=5&page=2 [7 July 2009].
Solomon, Z., Weissman, M., Levi, G., Fried, B., Mikolinsar, M., Benbenishty, R., Florian, V., & Bleich, A. 1992, 'From Front Line to Home Front: a Study of Secondary Traumatization', *Family Process*, vol. 31, no. 3, pp. 289–302.
Volkan, V. D. 2009, *The Next Chapter: Consequences of Societal Trauma*, unpublished manuscript.

Part I

"In the Terrible Silence That Followed"

Soldiers, Society, and Combat Stress Reaction

"Although we had moved on to other places, although we built other worlds for ourselves, in truth we all remained there, in the dissipating black smoke, in the terrible silence that followed, mute, each of us alone."

Menachem Ansbacher, *Fragment of the Silver Platter**

*Ansbacher (2007). Menachem Ansbacher was commander of the Tel Saki post in the Golan Heights during the Yom Kippur War.

1 Trapped in the Myth

A soldier goes to war. It is as though he has spent his entire life preparing for this moment. He knew that one day his turn would come. He would be called up for military service—regular or reserve—don his uniform, take his weapon in hand, and go off to that unknown about which he has heard so much. He bears a heavy burden: such responsibilities as "the fate of the nation" and those beliefs and myths—though they may be contested—in whose name he fights. He is weighted with expectations: those of his commanders, of the entire nation, and of himself, and with the hopes of his family, his friends, and his fellow soldiers. He carries with him as well concern for the family that he is leaving behind, the pain of separation, and fear of being killed, taken prisoner, or returning injured.

Soldiers are usually shielded from the full brunt of these concerns by an "illusion of safety," the faith, shared by most human beings, in their ability to overcome danger and difficulty. The army complements this illusion with training and equipment and by instilling in soldiers trust in their commanders, identification with their unit, and the sense of belonging to a group whose size and strength inspire confidence (Solomon 1993).[1] When the soldier finds himself engaged in prolonged battles, when he is exposed to harsh physical conditions and deprived of sleep and food, his faith in the protective mechanisms of the army weakens and the illusion of safety begins to erode. Indeed even in a brief military engagement, if a soldier faces the threat of imminent death, witnesses the deaths of comrades and commanders, finds himself in a situation of powerlessness, or finds his expectations undermined, the illusion of safety crumbles, and he is liable to suffer combat stress reaction (CSR) (Solomon 1993).

Attempts to identify traits that might make soldiers more prone to CSR or post-traumatic stress disorder (PTSD) have not yielded definitive findings. Based on the screening parameters currently in use, it appears to be exceedingly difficult, if not impossible, to make predictions of this kind (Zohar et al. 2009). Current knowledge suggests that every person has a breaking point, and whether one reaches that point depends on the intensity of the battle and the combined effects of an array of factors.

While the term "combat stress reaction" was coined in 1973, the condition had been observed and discussed under various names for centuries. During the European wars of the eighteenth century and the American Civil War, the phenomenon was referred to as "nostalgia," reflecting a belief that it was rooted in a longing for home. The terms "shell shock" and "battle shock" gained currency during World War I, a phrasing based on the notion that soldiers were experiencing a neurological reaction to shock waves from artillery shells. Later, under the influence of Freudian ideas, the syndrome came to be known as "war neurosis," which implied preexisting pathologies reawakened by war. During World War II the US military adopted the term "battle fatigue" in an attempt to confer upon the phenomenon the characteristics of physical exhaustion, which could be overcome with rest and good nutrition. Far from random, these terminological transformations reflect the evolution of the very understanding of trauma. The term commonly employed today, CSR, embodies a nonjudgmental attitude, founded on the understanding that the syndrome is the direct result of the events of battle, without limiting the condition's symptomology or scope.[2]

Through most of the twentieth century, those suffering from CSR were subject to condemnation and regarded as cowards, deserters, or mentally ill, despite developments, over the same period, in psychiatry and the study of emotional trauma. In Israel, authorities instituted sustained attempts to treat CSR only in the wake of the Yom Kippur War (1973). In the US the ongoing effects of CSR gained recognition from the psychiatric establishment only in 1980.[3] In retrospect it has become clear that all wars waged in Israel and elsewhere have produced large numbers of CSR sufferers and that the armies, though they denied the existence of the phenomenon and disregarded the plight of its victims, nevertheless collected information on it. This information gathering, however, did not lead to official recognition of CSR as a legitimate psychiatric syndrome, and thus research and therapeutic resources lagged. The information amassed in the course of each individual war was subsequently lost and forgotten, perhaps suppressed, while what therapeutic knowledge existed remained unimplemented, despite the fact that, as early as World War I, basic treatment methods had been developed that are still largely valid today.

Throughout the Western world, a similar process of belated recognition has characterized the historical development of attitudes toward CSR. Although only a handful of clinicians studied war trauma, the evidence was overwhelming. Meanwhile, military authorities, psychiatric professionals, and therapists remained indifferent to this mounting evidence for years. Today psychiatrists and clinicians regard this delay as a "historical professional error" (Levy et al. 1990).

Over the past two decades, Israel has witnessed major progress in the treatment of CSR and PTSD, and now serves as a model for other countries.[4] After the 1973 Yom Kippur War, military physicians and psychiatrists began compiling information on combat trauma, though this remained the unsystematic work of individuals until 1980, when the Israeli Defense Forces (IDF) established the Combat Stress Reactions Unit, a research unit dedicated exclusively to CSR. Charged with disseminating its findings on the diagnosis and treatment of CSR to field medical teams, the research unit was able to implement its work on a wide scale with the First Lebanon War in 1982 (known in Israel as "Operation Peace for the Galilee"). Despite this progress within the IDF in the treatment of CSR, nearly

20 years passed before the Defense Ministry began, in the late 1990s, to recognize the needs of veterans afflicted with PTSD. This change in policy was prompted by the activism of former prisoners of war, who organized an advocacy group, Erim Balayla ("Awake at Night"), and lobbied the Defense Ministry to identify PTSD victims among the population of former POWs.[5] Additional self-help groups and public advocacy organizations helped further raise public awareness on the issue.[6]

In response to pressure from these groups, and following protracted deliberation in the Labor, Welfare and Health Committee of the Israeli Parliament (the Knesset), in 2000 the Knesset passed a law acknowledging, for the first time, the unique character of CSR and PTSD among soldiers, differentiating these syndromes from preexisting forms of mental illness (*The Disability Law* 2000). According to Member of the Knesset (MK) Zahava Galon, who drafted the legislation, "for the first time a distinction is being made between people with mental illness and people who have been injured in battles to which they were sent on our behalf. Those afflicted with battle shock are not mentally ill." (Knesset Labor, Welfare and Health Committee 2000). Throughout the deliberations over the bill, MK Galon insisted on the importance of the law and the public legitimacy that it would confer on soldiers who "went to [. . .] battle mentally and physically healthy and returned injured." In doing so, Galon gave expression to the insight that social support for trauma victims, particularly those who experienced their trauma in the service of the nation, has both ethical and therapeutic value. Nevertheless, over a decade later this insight appears not to have been fully internalized by the Ministry of Defense, whose reports still place CSR under the category of mental illness, with just a note mentioning PTSD.[7] Traumatized soldiers continue to encounter distrust and disesteem by officials and medical committees when they seek diagnosis and pursue recognition as wounded veterans. Difficulty in accepting the phenomenon still prevails in the public view, as do the shame and feelings of guilt associated with it among traumatized soldiers, only a minority of whom seeks treatment. Moreover, recently, claims that trauma is being excessively legitimized have been heard in public discourse and even among psychiatrists, some of whom believe that Israel is moving "from a discourse of fighters to a discourse of victims."[8]

Another, relatively new topic came to the fore during the late 1980s, after the IDF's CSR unit had already been established. Israel's defense establishment was then encountering a type of traumatic event that it had never seen before, one that it still has trouble dealing with today. Soldiers were suffering trauma in the wake of events in which they themselves initiated the violence. This form of traumatic experience first garnered public attention as the conflict with the Palestinians escalated during the First Intifada, when the IDF's use of force against civilians rose to unprecedented levels. The moral and emotional impact on the soldiers of their service in the Occupied Territories, and the question of whether these soldiers are actually traumatized or "merely" afflicted with profound feelings of guilt, continue to elicit emotional and vigorous debate among Israelis. The clamor and controversy are often reminiscent of the profound denial of CSR and PTSD that characterized the early decades of Israel's statehood.

The state's attitudes toward soldiers traumatized by war are shaped by a set of tensions. On the one hand, the military establishment needs to preserve its character as a fighting force that cultivates courage and expects soldiers to place themselves unhesitatingly in the line of fire. At the same time, the state has a moral duty to acknowledge the personal suffering of the wounded—including the psychologically wounded—and the military establishment and society as a whole bear the responsibility for the price paid by the individual in service to the state. The position, image, and expectations of the soldier are characterized by contradictory impulses within the societies that send him into battle: adoration, on the one hand, and the expectation of total sacrifice and absence of personal needs, on the other.

In Israel, despite certain gestures of cultural, social, and financial support, such as national ceremonies or special rights afforded to demobilized combat soldiers, the state's relations with its soldiers is generally marked by ambivalence. While in official rhetoric soldiers are held in high esteem, very often their practical needs are not met.[9] Soldiers and their families often articulate dissatisfaction and disappointment with this gap between rhetoric and reality (Witztum & Malkinson 1993). In fact, the official admiration for the soldier is something of a double-edged sword: the soldier is placed on a pedestal as an example to the nation and showered with love and esteem. Yet from this lofty position, he cannot display pain, weakness, or doubt. Society traps its soldiers within a myth that, however elevated the language in which it is expressed, hinders the expression of individual pain, fear, or insecurity. In the words of Menachem Ansbacher, commander of the Tel Saki post in the Golan Heights during the Yom Kippur War,

> Heroic paratroopers don't need anything. They are either immune to harm or dead. Anything in between is just a matter of bodywork and a fresh paint-job. Scratches on the interior or hidden structural damage? Those are things that a paratrooper is supposed to deal with himself. Heroes can bleed for ten or twenty years. That's part of the contract. A lifelong contract.
>
> (Ansbacher 2007, p. 13)

Imprisoned by a myth, soldiers find the walls especially imposing when the war in which they participate is controversial. In such wars, one segment of the public regards soldiers as the nation's saviors and expects of them heroism, determination, and a constant mobilization of all of their mental and physical resources, without the smallest expression of doubt. Another segment rejects the official, heroic image of the soldier, while often showing hostility toward individual soldiers, seeing them as enforcers of a policy that they repudiate.

When the drums of war stop beating and the soldiers come home, the struggle to reintegrate into everyday life begins. Some feel detached and must undergo a process of emotional reorganization. Others experience a sense of detachment, a disconnect from the collective whose lives seemingly went on as usual, while those who fought on the nation's behalf often find themselves beset with emotional, physical, and financial difficulties. Reservists, for example, who constitute an essential part of the IDF's forces, especially during war, must recoup losses or deal with financial hardships from missed work on their own when they return from their service. For soldiers wounded in war, the struggles of returning to daily life are exponentially compounded, as their lives will never be the same. Those who have suffered psychological injury may even endure additional trauma while attempting to reintegrate. The peculiar behavior of the traumatized soldier is often met with misunderstanding by his coworkers, family, and community, and instead of a hero he finds himself the object of suspicion, exacerbating the problem. This additional trauma, compounding the original one, often further hinders the prospects of recovery. The very invisibility of the bloodless wound complicates the wounded veteran's interactions with those involved in the recovery process, from family and friends to coworkers and representatives of government agencies. Familial and communal relationships of the traumatized soldier are invariably transformed, now marked by stress and tensions. While the soldier often feels that nobody can understand him, his family experiences disappointment brought on by his unfamiliar behavior.

Because in Israel people live with a constant security threat, when a war ends or a terror attack is over, a great effort is made—by the state and by individuals—to put things "back on track" as quickly as possible in an attempt to conduct normal civilian life under the shadow of constant alert. A byproduct of this emphasis on quickly returning to normal life includes the public silencing of any discussion about the price of war in general, and its emotional cost in particular. An expectation exists as well that returning soldiers will put the war behind, rather than turning their experiences into a personal crisis or allowing themselves to be overly affected by what they've just been through. This silencing of discussion about the price of war in Israel should not be seen as incompatible with the fact that war and security threats constitute a prominent part of Israeli public discourse, even in periods of calm. On the contrary, ignoring the price of war fortifies the prevalent belief in the inevitability of war and the intractability of the Israeli-Palestinian conflict. These beliefs, political psychologist Daniel Bar-Tal suggests, function as defense mechanisms that enable Israelis to live with the persistent threat of war hovering over them.[10] But these beliefs trap Israeli society in a perpetual discourse on war-as-fate, propping up the myths of siege, heroism, and defense. These patterns encumber legitimization of the problems encountered by war veterans, especially the psychologically impaired, who allegedly fail to meet the norm of "normalizing" the war.

Haim Dasberg argues that none of the existing theoretical models of trauma take into account the fact that victims of organized violence—soldiers among them—suffer from a form of social pathology to which society reacts with a corresponding pathology of its own. The two pathologies generate a negative and intensifying reciprocal effect. Dasberg proposes that in some instances the term "post-traumatic stress disorder" be replaced by "post-organized-violence disorder" which, in his view, also encompasses the fraught interactions that arise between victims of organized violence and their families and communities (Dasberg 1987).

The foregoing points to the need for a new understanding, however difficult to accept, regarding society's attitudes toward those who fight on its behalf. Soldiers are cast in a multifaceted role. They are the nation's defenders and heroes, but also victims of the violence that they themselves help perpetrate. They are sent by the nation to safeguard what is perceived as a supreme common interest, and while doing so they experience violence and danger, both as defenders and as aggressors. On their return, they frequently encounter indifference and even criticism concerning how the war was waged or their own reaction to it.

Notes

1. The term "illusion of safety" was coined by the American military psychiatrist Jon Shaw (Solomon 1993).
2. On how the naming of the phenomenon evolved, see Bleich (1990); Solomon (1993), Chap. 3.
3. As noted in the introduction, that was the first year in which PTSD appeared in the American Psychiatric Association's *Diagnostic and Statistical Manual of Mental Disorders* as a separate syndrome, one precipitated by an external event rather than by a prior mental disorder. Defining the kinds of events associated with PTSD made it possible to recognize CSR as a syndrome and events in battle as the cause of trauma (Blank 1985).
4. Author's interview with Prof. Avi Bleich, former head of the IDF Mental Health Department and currently director of Lev-Hasharon Medical Center and chair of NATAL's professional steering committee, January 2009.
5. Author's interview with Miri Shalit, director of Rehabilitation Services in the Dan District, the Rehabilitation Division, 17 February 2009. The group in question went on to form the *Erim Balayla* ("Awake at Night") association.
6. For example, the Families of Shell-Shock Victims association, whose chair, Pirha Goldstein, participated in the legislative deliberations and continued the struggle on behalf of the law's implementation. See Sinai (2001).
7. See the statement of Defense Ministry Director General Pinchas Buchris (especially Slide No. 11 in the presentation), and that of the director of the Defense Ministry's Disabled Rehabilitation Division, Kuti Mor (particularly slides 8 and 9 in the presentation), before the Public Committee to Assess Eligibility for Assistance from the Rehabilitation Divisions, 2010 (Goren Committee). The committee deliberations and the statements of those who appeared before it are available to the public at the following site: www.vaadatgoren.gov.il. Retrieved on 2 April 2010. (Hebrew)
8. Author's interview with Prof. Avi Bleich, September 2008.
9. For example, compensation for reserve soldiers for the loss of working days does not cover the real loss; reservists who are students often complain about the army's inflexibility with their service dates and unwillingness to accommodate their class schedules; wounded soldiers face huge difficulties getting the compensation and treatments they require.
10. On the societal beliefs that make living with the conflict possible, see Bar-Tal (2007).

References

Ansbacher, M. 2007, *Fragment of the Silver Platter*, Daniella De-Nur, Tel Aviv. (Hebrew)

Bar-Tal, D. 2007, *Living with the Conflict, Socio-Psychological Analysis of the Jewish Society in Israel*, Carmel, Jerusalem. (Hebrew)

Blank, A. S. 1985, 'The Veterans Administration's Vietnam Veterans Outreach and Counseling Centers' in *The Trauma of War: Stress and Recovery in Viet Nam Veterans*, eds S. M. Sonnenberg, A. S. Blank, & J. A. Talbott, American Psychiatric Press, Washington, DC, Chapter 11, pp. 229–238.

Bleich, A. 1990, 'Acute Combat Stress Reaction: Pathogenic, Diagnostic and Therapeutic Aspects', *I.D.F. Medical Corps Bulletin*, vol. 32, pp. 43–45. (Hebrew)
Bleich, A. 2000, 'Military Psychiatry in Israel: a 50-Year Perspective', *Harefuah*, vol. 138, no. 9, pp. 728–733.
Dasberg, H. 1987, 'Israeli Society vis-à-vis Organized Trauma, or the Therapist vis-à-vis the Survivor' in *Sichot*, vol. 1, no. 2, pp. 98–103. (Hebrew)
The Disability Law (Benefits and Rehabilitation), Amendment No. 21 (Psychological Disability and Battle Shock), 2000, Israel.
Israel, Knesset Labor, Welfare and Health Committee, Protocol No. 125, 23 May 2000.
Levy, A., Witztum, E., Granek, M., & Kotler, M. 1990, 'The Treatment of Combat Stress Reaction in the IDF, 1948–1973', *Harefuah*, vol. 32, pp. 49–53.
Sinai, R. 2001, 'They Did Not Run Away', *Haaretz* (English edition), 20 September.
Solomon, Z. 1993, *Combat Stress Reaction, the Enduring Toll of War*, Plenum Press, New York.
Witztum, E., & Malkinson, R. 1993, 'Bereavement and Memorialization: the Two Faces of the National Myth' in *Loss and Bereavement in Jewish Society in Israel*, eds E. Witztum & R. Malkinson, Kanah and the Ministry of Defense, Tel Aviv, pp. 231–258. (Hebrew)
Zohar, J., Fostick, L., Cohen, A., Bleich, A., Dolfin, D., Weissman, Z., Doron, M., Kaplan, Z., Klein, E., & Shalev, A. 2009, 'Risk Factors for the Development of Post-Traumatic Stress Disorder following Combat Trauma: a Semiprospective Study', *Journal of Clinical Psychiatry*, vol. 70, no. 12, pp. 1629–1635.

2 The Starting Point

World War I: The Test of Loyalty and the Myth of the War Experience

> On November 9, 1914, a French cobbler from Arques, a small village some 25 miles from the warfront in Belgium, came upon Lance-Sergeant William Walton, a 26-year-old British soldier, wounded in his left arm and suffering from a heavy cough, hunger, and fatigue. The cobbler took pity on the soldier, debilitated by four months of combat in some of the bloodiest battles of the war. He took Walton into his home and shared the only bed he owned. According to the cobbler's testimony, Walton remained in his house in a state of shock and confusion for two months. Sometimes he would go out into the village and talk with British soldiers stationed there. On these occasions, he gave no appearance of trying to conceal himself or his identity. On March 3, Walton was arrested by the French military police, handed over to British military authorities, and tried by court martial for desertion. A senior officer in the division who discerned Walton's troubled emotional state asked that he be sent for medical evaluation, but no attention was paid to his request. On March 23, 1915, Lance-Sergeant Walton was executed by firing squad.[1]

Lance-Sergeant Walton's story was not unusual. Interminable bloody battles in which millions were killed and wounded, and the appalling conditions of trench warfare, left hundreds of thousands of soldiers psychologically injured. Psychologically traumatized soldiers, however, were regarded as psychopaths, deserters, and cowards, who placed their own interests above the common good (Brunner 1991). This disparaging view of trauma victims and the punitive measures for dealing with them were shared by all of the armies involved in the conflict. Although as early as the eighteenth century an Austrian physician had noted the inefficacy of sanctions or threats in mitigating the phenomenon then known as "nostalgia," militaries chose to ignore the growing understanding of the problem's medical characteristics and kept treating sufferers with suspicion or outright hostility (Levy et al. 1989).

Most physicians in Austria-Hungary during World War I viewed their primary task as facilitating the rapid return of wounded soldiers to combat. In pursuit of this goal, they regularly employed violent therapeutic methods, such as electric shocks of increasing voltage. Often reaching "an unbearable point", these electroshock treatments occasionally resulted in death or drove patients to suicide (Babington 1997, pp. 65–66).[2] These practices were based on the assumption that traumatized soldiers "fled from the war into treatment", and therefore implemented a policy, which combined hours of painful electric shocks with strict military discipline, and an atmosphere of "unquestioning, unreasoning obedience".[3] This was aimed at compelling the soldiers to return to their units, as the conditions in the hospital were more unbearable than those in the front. In 1916 the German Society for Psychiatry officially declared that its members never forget "that we physicians have now to put all our work in the service of one mission: to serve our army and our fatherland" (quoted in Brunner 2002). They saw their duty as primarily to "fill the ranks" of the front line rather than to provide care to injured soldiers. Most German psychiatrists during this period referred to the phenomenon of war-induced psychological trauma as a "disease of the will," regarding it, at best, as a soldier's unconscious attempt to escape his duties, though more often it was seen as deliberate malingering, or *Rentenkampfhysteria* ("hysteria to secure a pension"), a ploy to obtain compensation from the state. Obviously when physicians prioritize the needs of the military over those of their patients, they disregard symptoms and arrive at a convenient etiology: sufferers are malingerers and are undeserving of a discharge with financial compensation. Even those psychiatrists who opposed censuring traumatized soldiers or categorizing "war neurosis," as it was known during World War I, as hysteria did so out of ideology rather than professional conviction. They feared that any identification of war neurosis with hysteria would disgrace the army and thereby harm the fatherland (Brunner 2002).

As the story of Lance-Sergeant Walton shows, these attitudes were not unique to Germany and Austria. During the war, the British army executed 18 soldiers for "cowardice," and another 266 for desertion. Within a few years of the close of the war, the British public began to raise concerns that many of those who had been executed on these two charges had merely suffered from "shell shock," finally leading to new legislation that abolished the death penalty for "cowardice" and instead set penal servitude as the punishment for desertion (Babington 1997). In war, loyalty is a supreme value, and in the case of soldiers psychologically traumatized during World War I, we see a double failure to live up to this ideal: on the one hand, the loyalty of these soldiers to their homelands was called into doubt; on the other, their commanders and doctors shirked the duty of loyalty they owed to the soldiers, forsaking them in favor of ideological considerations.

With World War I, what historian George Mosse has called the "Myth of the War Experience" (Mosse 1990), the idea of war as a profoundly meaningful, even sacred event, reached its apotheosis in Europe. The roots of this myth reach back to the late eighteenth and early nineteenth centuries. Until that point, war had been largely a struggle between rival monarchies, but with the French Revolution and the wars of German unification, fundamental changes occurred in the nature of warfare and the composition of European armies (Mosse 1990). Armies no longer consisted principally of hooligans and vagabonds, mercenaries and forced conscripts. Many soldiers voluntarily enlisted in the French Revolutionary Army, inspired by the ideals of the revolution and the defense of France. They tended to be young, educated, and middle-class. The figure of the soldier became idealized and adored in the national consciousness of Revolutionary France. The Myth of the War Experience emerged concomitantly with this new type of soldier, transforming prevailing attitudes toward war, society's expectations of soldiers, and soldiers' expectations of themselves. The myth glorified self-sacrifice and camaraderie, and elevated war to a symbol of masculinity, personal renewal, and national revival. Within this ideological climate, war came to be seen as a sacred experience, an expression of the shared will of the people.

In the early twentieth century, a contradictory set of attitudes toward war emerged: on the one hand, war came to be seen as an outlet for patriotism and the culmination of a quest for meaning, both personal and collective. On the other hand, war came to be seen as a theater of adventure where an idealized masculine hero could perform courageous deeds. According to Mosse, young men of the era viewed war as the greatest human drama in which they could participate, while the common soldier was glorified as the "New Man" and national savior (Mosse 1990). These attitudes enabled soldiers to believe that they could collectively confront death, elevating war to the loftiest sphere. On the eve of World War I, the desire to pass what had come to be seen as a test of masculinity in the crucible of war could be found among many of the young men of Europe.

But then the war started. It turned into a massacre, one wholly inconsistent with the glorified image of war: people lost their lives in inconceivable numbers and suffered horrifying injuries.[4] With no end in sight, soldiers experienced distress and fear that contrasted jarringly with the enthusiasm that had carried them to war in the first place. In the face of such devastation and disappointment, the authorities and architects of the war did not, of course, renounce the war but rather sought to resolve the contradictions by glorifying the fallen soldiers and reinforcing the myth. This also meant vilifying those suffering with invisible wounds.

The very sociocultural processes that had shaped the attitudes toward war in Europe in the lead-up to World War I also hampered recognition of CSR. Such recognition would have undermined the war ideal and revealed the horrors obscured by the Myth of the War Experience. The all-too-human symptoms of CSR stand in stark contrast to the myth of masculinity, according to which soldiers are creatures of utter selflessness, fortitude, and patriotism, a buttress against personal weakness and difficulties. CSR contradicts the ideals of strength, heroism, and the mythic image of the military. The steadfastness of a soldier—and even more so, that of a commanding officer—must be such that he "neither fears, nor cries, nor experiences hunger, cold or fatigue" (Ansbacher 2007, p. 29).

Learning and Forgetting: Between the Two World Wars

Although CSR was widely observed and discussed during World War I, trauma research was then in its infancy, and psychiatric clinicians proved reluctant to acknowledge it. On the other hand, a psychoanalytic understanding of CSR began to emerge even before the conclusion of the war.[5] Prevailing theories of "shell shock" began to give way to a psychoanalytic theory of "war stress." The latter held that the events of war could indeed cause serious psychological disturbances, memories of which could inflict lifelong torment.

In England, two years after the armistice, 65,000 soldiers were recognized as psychiatric war casualties. By 1939 this number had grown to 120,000 recipients of psychiatric casualty pensions. In the US Army about 20%, or some 220,000, of the 1,130,000 troops who served in Europe were hospitalized and treated in psychiatric facilities during World War I. The sheer force of these numbers led, for the first time in world medical history, to an acceptance of the idea that psychological trauma can cause prolonged disturbances and thus long-term psychological disability (Witztum 2002).[6] Toward the end of World War I, the PIE Principles (proximity, immediacy, expectancy), formulated by US chief of army psychiatry Thomas W. Salmon, came into use as the treatment guidelines for CSR (then called shell shock or war neurosis) (Levy et al. 1989).[7] Soldiers would undergo treatment as soon as possible after the first onset of symptoms. The actual treatment was based on rest, good food, and relatively simple forms of supportive psychotherapy, aimed at instilling optimism and characterized by persuasion and suggestion. Some estimations proclaim that 65% of recipients reached a quick recovery. Unfortunately, the treatment was practiced on a small scale and could not help those who did not enjoy a speedy recovery and were therefore sent home (probably developing PTSD, which was not yet understood as such) (Pols & Oak 2007). Salmon's principles still form the basic rules for the treatment of CSR. For a moment, it seemed as though the mental health community had succeeded in overcoming its ideological biases.

However, over the two decades between the two World Wars, the knowledge amassed on CSR all but disappeared. On the eve of America's entry into World War II, the US Army had no preparations in place for the care of CSR victims, regarding the issue as marginal. No one was trained to care for the psychologically traumatized, there existed no appropriate channels for reporting instances of trauma, and in 1941 psychiatrists were actually discharged from the military due to budget cuts (Solomon 1995). During the first years of World War II the army abandoned Salmon's ideas, which had come to seem irrelevant since military and psychiatric leaders now believed they could screen soldiers for vulnerability to psychiatric disorders (Pols & Oak 2007).

It quickly became clear, however, that CSR was not a one-time phenomenon confined to World War I. In the British army, for example, the proportion of psychologically wounded within the entire wounded population ranged from 2% to 30% over the course of the war, depending on the type of combat (Babington 1997). The number of CSR cases in the American army was so high that Chief of Staff George Marshall complained in 1943 that "the number of soldiers being discharged from the army on psychiatric grounds was greater than the number being inducted" (Babington 1997, p. 151).[8] With psychological trauma so prevalent, the Americans were forced to recall psychiatrists to military duty and pursue treatment methods.

Yet even with these developments, the military continued to deny the true nature of CSR. The treatments developed by American military psychiatrists affirmed the old paradigm by which CSR was seen as a passing phenomenon rooted in a victim's preexisting personality. The very notion of a post-traumatic stress disorder caused by the events of war contradicted one of the fundamental assumptions of psychoanalysis of that period—namely, that the effects of trauma can be profound and prolonged only when the trauma occurs during childhood (Boulander 1985). The common Freudian treatment for what analysts called "war neurosis" was long-term psychoanalysis. The American military establishment became concerned that an epidemic was in the making. General Omar Bradley gave the orders to rename the condition "battle fatigue" or "battle exhaustion," with a corresponding directive to grant those afflicted a week's leave (Bleich 1990; Solomon 1993). This decision, consistent with an understanding of the syndrome as a passing disturbance with no long-term consequences, diverted attention to the physical and generally more easily addressed features of the syndrome, symptoms that could be treated through rest and proper nutrition. The fact that the name change came by military fiat rather than from medical professional channels points to the sense of panic over the potential ramifications of CSR for soldier morale. Nevertheless, the syndrome's direct linkage to the combat experience heralded a change in official attitude toward CSR sufferers. In this sense General Bradley's decision may be seen as an important step toward ending the de-legitimization of those afflicted with CSR. Rather than denouncing them as cowards and shirkers, or accusing them of weaknesses of character, the military establishment recognized these soldiers' exhaustion and need for treatment, albeit only at a physical level.

This flawed perspective on psychological trauma had a profound and adverse impact on the treatment of Holocaust survivors after the war. Eliezer Witztum relates appalling instances in which American psychiatrists dismissed survivors' accounts of psychological symptoms, attributing these to preexisting psychological disorders (Witztum 2002). Rather than the actual psychological health of the survivors, this attitude signaled the reluctance of clinicians to reconsider their approach and the external biases that influenced the field of trauma research.

The phenomenon of soldiers with no visible injuries suffering from clinical symptoms of acute anxiety, limb paralysis, blindness, deafness, confusion, and serious cognitive and memory disturbances did generate considerable interest within the mental health community from World War I on (Witztum 2002).[9] However, this interest was invariably intertwined with political, economic, and military considerations and at that time produced no medical treatment capable of helping CSR sufferers.

Since its infancy, the field of psychological trauma research has been a locus of conflicting ideologies and interests. Suspicions of deception have always hovered over trauma victims like a dark cloud. The main reason for this, according to José Brunner, is that, unlike most psychological disturbances, the core experience that gives rise to trauma lies within a defined external reality (Brunner 2002). If an external event can be isolated and identified as having directly caused trauma, then it follows that someone bears the responsibility. This implication of blame has always been a source of contention: it can lead victims to demand compensation, while those held responsible try to renounce accountability.

Such was the case with railroad and industrial accidents that became increasingly common during the nineteenth century. Such accidents came to be seen as prime causes of traumatic disorders among civilians, and as soon as passengers and workers had the opportunity to pursue legal action and claim damages, doctors were brought in. Legal wrangling over compensation for injuries necessitated the services of clinicians capable of testifying to the presence or absence of psychological trauma. Psychiatrists would sometimes represent claimants, sometimes companies—in which case, their purpose was to protect their employers from the need to pay compensation (Brunner 2002). Psychiatric professional discourse became tainted by financial considerations, and the expert opinions of clinicians depended on who had hired them—the plaintiff or the defendant. Thus, despite the emerging theoretical frameworks developed to address trauma, many psychiatrists continued to deny the existence of post-traumatic effects, portraying the entire syndrome as a sham aimed at securing compensation (Witztum 2002). The difficulty in identifying psychological trauma, whose long-term symptoms often manifest after a delay and may seem out of proportion to the traumatic event, reinforced these suspicions of fraud.

Identifying CSR, a special type of psychological trauma, presents a further set of complications, which lie primarily in the chaotic nature of war. The behavior of the injured can seem, at first glance, like a reasonable response to an unreasonable situation. For a soldier overcome with paralyzing fear when faced with the expectation of walking into the line of fire, this sounds like a "normal" reaction rather than a disorder of a wounded mind. When PTSD is delayed in onset—appearing only after the soldier has returned, seemingly healthy, from his military service—diagnosis and recognition become harder still (Solomon 1993; Solomon et al. 1994).

When one considers the conditions of warfare, I think what is harder to believe than the existence of CSR is the fact that more soldiers do not suffer from it, instead adapting to their unreasonable situation and coping with the stresses of war unimpaired by mental injury. This fact in itself makes it even harder to sympathize with the psychologically traumatized. Moreover, prejudicial attitudes toward CSR sufferers may also be rooted in the fact that an intense existential fear lies at the syndrome's core, a fear that saps one's ability to continue fighting.

All soldiers in combat face a profound unconscious and involuntary quandary—whether to fight or flee—a conflict between the instinct for self-preservation and the demands of one's duty (Bleich 1990; Pols & Oak 2007). Of course other factors contribute to whether this unconscious conflict—shared by all soldiers in battle—is exacerbated and manifests in CSR. However, outsiders, and certainly those who have not taken part in combat, find it difficult, if not impossible, to understand the breakdown experienced by the soldier under extreme and continuous menace.

Prejudices persist, and suspicions that victims of PTSD are feigning illness in order to obtain compensation remain prevalent even today. Although the number of malingerers has been shown time and again to be exceedingly small, many of those afflicted with psychological trauma continue to be treated with suspicion and labeled as "fraudulent claimants" (Litman 2007).[10]

Notes

1. The entire incident, documented in official British military history, is recounted in Babington (1997).
2. The quotation in Babington (1997) is from a memorandum by Sigmund Freud, "The Electrical Treatment of War Neurosis," submitted during World War I, per an invitation by the Austrian War Ministry, who set up an inquiry on this issue after the war.
3. 'Notes from German and Austrian Medical Journal, Disciplinary Treatment of Shell-Shock', *British Medical Journal*, 1916, vol. 2, p. 882, quoted in Babington, 1997, p. 65. The German journal published the original account of Dr. Kaufman, who was responsible for this treatment in a German army hospital next to the front.
4. Casualty estimates for the war point to some 16 million fatalities, 10 million of them soldiers, and to 21 million wounded (soldiers and civilians).
5. On the development of these approaches see Brunner (1991).
6. See also the explanation of the types of psychiatric disability that determine eligibility for UK war disablement pensions.
7. Thomas Williams Salmon was chief of army psychiatry for the American Expeditionary Forces in World War I. The PIE Principles that he formulated are as follows: *proximity*—treat the casualties as close to the battlefront as possible; *immediacy*—treat them without delay; *expectation*—send a clear therapeutic message that the soldier's symptoms are merely a temporary "reaction" and that he is expected to recover and return to duty. On Salmon's contribution to the development of treatment for CSR sufferers (then referred to as "shell shock"), see Ozarin (2002).
8. For prevalence of psychological trauma among US soldiers, see Witztum (2002). According to the data presented by Witztum, a million soldiers were hospitalized for psychiatric disturbances.
9. Witztum cites data pointing to some 1,100 publications on the topic during 1914–1919.
10. Litman quotes the late Dr. Y. Avni, who called such claimants *pitzuyentim* ("seekers of compensation") rather than *patzyentim* ("patients").

References

Ansbacher, M. 2007, *Fragment of the Silver Platter*, Daniella De-Nur, Tel Aviv. (Hebrew)

Babington, A. 1997, *Shell Shock, a History of the Changing Attitudes to War Neurosis*, L. Cooper, London.

Bleich, A. 1990, 'Acute Combat Stress Reaction: Pathogenic, Diagnostic and Therapeutic Aspects', *I.D.F. Medical Corps Bulletin*, vol. 32, pp. 43–45. (Hebrew)

Boulanger, G. 1985, 'Post Traumatic Stress Disorder: an Old Problem with a New Name' in *The Trauma of War: Stress and Recovery in Viet Nam Veterans*, eds. S. M. Sonnenberg, A. S. Blank, & J. A. Talbott, American Psychiatric Press, Washington, D.C., pp. 13–29.

Brunner, J. 1991, 'Psychiatry, Psychoanalysis and Politics during the First World War', *Journal of the History of the Behavioral Sciences*, vol. 27, pp. 353–365.

Brunner, J. 2002, 'Identifications, Suspicions and the History of Traumatic Disorders', *Harvard Review of Psychiatry*, vol. 10, no. 3, pp. 179–184.

Levy, A., Witztum, E., Granek, M., & Kotler, M. 1989, 'Combat Reactions in Israel's Wars, 1948–1973, Part 1: General Background and History, Methodology and a Review of the Literature of the Period', *Sichot*, vol. 4, no. 1, pp. 60–70. (Hebrew)

Litman, S. 2007, Editor's note on the article by A. Bleich & Y. Melamed, 'Post-Traumatic Psychological Impairment Subsequent to Military Service', *Refuah vMishpat* [Law and Medicine], vol. 37, p. 44. (Hebrew)

Mosse, G. 1990, *Fallen Soldiers: Reshaping the Memory of the World Wars*, Oxford University Press, New York.

Ozarin, L. 2002, 'Thomas William Salmon: Psychiatry in Time of War', *Psychiatric News*, vol. 37, no. 13, p. 38.

Pols, H., & Oak, S. 2007, 'WAR & Military Mental Health: the US Psychiatric Response in the 20th Century', *American Journal of Public Health*, vol. 97, no. 12, pp. 2132–2142.

Solomon, Z. 1993, *Combat Stress Reaction, the Enduring Toll of War*, Plenum Press, New York.

Solomon, Z. 1995, 'Oscillating between Denial and Recognition of PTSD: Why Are Lessons Learned and Forgotten?', *Journal of Traumatic Stress*, vol. 8, no. 2, pp. 217–282.

Solomon, Z., Benbenishty, R., Waysman, M., & Bleich, A. 1994, 'The Role of Compensation in Rehabilitating Combat Stress Reaction Sufferers: a Weakening or Strengthening Factor?', *Harefuah*, vol. 127, pp. 450–455. (Hebrew)

Witztum, E. 2002, 'A History of the Concept of Psychological Disability' in *Mental Disability: Medical, Research Social, Legal and Rehabilitative Aspects*, eds. A. Bleich & Z. Solomon, Ministry of Defense, Tel Aviv, pp. 11–25. (Hebrew)

3 The Early Decades

Starting Point to Turning Point

Denial

They were called "*degim*"—degenerates, shirkers. Their fellow soldiers dissociated themselves from them during battle, and most continued to do so even 50 years later: "I'm not aware of one single case of battle shock [. . .] There were no such instances. Absolutely not [. . .] I do know of shirkers, people who were just cowardly and fled the fighting. That's all. No battle shock."[1] Physicians and psychiatrists also viewed them as weaklings, lacking in ideological fervor, who, conscripted in response to wartime needs, had not been reared in a spirit of pioneering and self-sacrifice and were therefore given to CSR (Heilperin 1949; Keynan 1998).

During the War of Independence, the newly founded state of Israel faced a conflict whose scope, duration, and intensity have been compared by Emmanuel Sivan to that of World War I (Sivan 1991). The country's per-population death rate was comparable to that of France, the country that suffered the greatest number of losses in WWI. Many Israelis instinctively shared this feeling at the time. The news of more and more fallen soldiers, the siege of Jerusalem, costly battles that, for a considerable period, brought no strategic advantage—all compounded the difficulty of coping with a long, exhausting war. In fact, in the midst of the war, Israelis noted similarities with WWI, particularly regarding the issue of severe psychological reactions to combat. Author Yeshurun Keshet, in his journal, compared the "unsettling desolation [. . .] of Jerusalem under bombardment" to the "melancholy that soldiers complained of" in the trenches (quoted in Sivan 1991, p. 21). A soldier wrote home from the front:

> Read *All Quiet on the Western Front* carefully, and you'll see that, if the location and conditions are changed, a fair number of the military and psychological descriptions are remarkably similar to the conditions that prevail here . . . especially from a psychological point of view. I assure you that you've never seen as many dead people as I've pulled off the ground, and that's something that numbs a person's emotions . . . It reaches the point where even when friends are killed beside me I find it hard—literally—to view it from any other perspective than that of the military loss, and I assure you that my own symptoms are by no means exceptionally severe.
>
> (quoted in Sivan 1991, p. 21)

Just three years after the Holocaust, pervasive fears that the fledgling state would be vanquished in its first battle for survival took on special meaning. The prevailing perception among Israelis at the time was that this was a war of "the few against the many," and this view profoundly influenced how people coped with violence and hardship.[2] The myths of heroism and sacrifice, cultivated in pre-state Israel from the time of the Jewish national awakening, when compounded by the experience of an acute immediate threat, generated psychological rejection of anything that could be perceived as weakness or potentially damaging to the prospects of victory. This is unquestionably one of the reasons why the number of traumatized soldiers in the War of Independence, including members of elite units, was completely undocumented by the IDF. Condemnation of CSR sufferers in the War of Independence was unequivocal. So far as can be ascertained, they received no treatment, and the entire issue was hushed up (Levy et al. 1989).

Another factor contributing to this sweeping denial of CSR can be found in attitudes commonly held by certain segments of the Palmach generation—that is, Israelis born between 1923 and 1930—whose ages ranged between 17 and 24 when the war broke out. This generation takes its name from the Palmach, the elite combat unit of the Hagannah, the largest of the three Jewish undergrounds, which would become the backbone of the IDF. The *sabras*, native-born Israelis, within this generation had been imbued with a sense of personal responsibility for the fate of the nation, educated and trained for heroism and sacrifice. From their personal writings and letters, one gets the sense that they identified completely with the national ethos on which they had been raised. While members of the older, founding generation expressed fears that those who grew up in pre-state Israel were spoiled and, in the hour of need, would fail to realize the hopes invested in them, the *sabras* readily embraced the role of the martyr, voluntarily and altruistically sacrificing themselves for the good of the nation (Almog 1998). They felt that the fate of Israel rested on their shoulders, and they bore this burden in solitude, virtually alone: "We've been left so alone," wrote Netiva Ben Yehuda, a *sabra* and renowned author who fought with the Palmach in the War of Independence (quoted in Sivan 1991, p. 62).

Native-born Jews were a very young demographic in Israel: during the War of Independence, over 70% of the *sabra* population was under conscription age (Sivan 1991). *Sabras* constituted a third of the fighting force, corresponding to their share of the 800,000 Jewish citizens of the newborn state, though they tended to serve as officers in greater numbers (Yablonka n.d.). The sacrifice made by those *sabras* old enough to fight indeed proved great, particularly in the early months of the war. Although by the armistice in 1949, casualties in this group corresponded proportionally to their numbers in service, *sabras* accounted for 45% of the dead during the first two months and 37% by the declaration of statehood and subsequent general mobilization. The blow that the *sabras* suffered as a group left a deep psychological imprint. It made them tougher and withdrawn, and strengthened their belief in the need for uncompromising self-sacrifice. They became unwilling to accept any form of weakness. This generational scar amplified the demands on the individual and precluded any show of consideration for those who fell short of expectations.

The *sabras* generally accepted as part of their generational group the foreign-born Jews who had grown up in pre-state Israel—that is, those who had immigrated before 1939. Like their *sabra* counterparts, these immigrants often served in command positions in the quasi-military pre-state organizations, and shared the ethos of self-sacrifice. Among this group, at least half who died in battle in the War on Independence had been ten years old or younger when they immigrated to pre-state Israel. They were thus *sabra* by education if not by birth, and had been socialized by the same educational frameworks as their native-born peers (Sivan 1991). Many of them embraced the values and ethos of the Yishuv even more resolutely than the *sabras* themselves. Even among those who had immigrated just a few years prior to being conscripted, quite a few exhibited the same dismissive attitude toward anyone who failed to meet the standards of the "New Jew."[3]

Periods of collective distress cultivate national myths and the need to foster collective fortitude. The individual's commitment to the demands of the collective and his or her belief in the necessity and justice of national goals can become so strong that the prospect of self-sacrifice appears natural, obvious, and even, at times, a privilege. Although not everyone felt the same absolute commitment to the needs of the nation, this worldview dominated the rhetoric and frame of mind. Oz Almog notes that desertion and evasion of duty were rare in the Palmach and met with harsh denunciation. Most soldiers exhibited a sense of intertwined personal and national obligation to persevere. Almog quotes an essay written by a soldier during the war:

> We are fighting all the way and we know what for and why . . . If our boys are fighting, they're doing it because they have to fight . . . because that's how it has to be with us. They can't disappoint their people—those who suffered and dreamed in the past and who died in misery.
>
> (S. Smargad, "That's How It Has to Be with Us: A Portrait of Our Youth," quoted in Almog 1998, p. 113)

The founding generation expressed deep gratitude for the way the *sabras* conducted themselves during the war, crowning them with heroes' laurels and showering them with love and esteem.[4] Even bereaved parents saw a dimension of justice in their misfortune and reconciled themselves to the loss of their children, mythical figures who, in their eyes, had avenged a history of abominations, had "finish[ed] the war against the Hellenizers."[5] Heroism and self-sacrifice permeated the post-war atmosphere. Individuals seen to personify these traits were celebrated, while anything or anyone deemed incompatible with them was condemned.

Although testimonies collected years later affirm the existence of numerous psychological casualties during the war, commanders in the field, who were the only ones responsible for identifying traumatized soldiers, effectively failed to do so (Levy et al. 1990). Military psychiatric units established on the home front—in Jaffa, Tzrifin, and Haifa—offered some treatment, but lacked uniform methods and made few efforts to return the recovered patients to service, based on Salmon's principles of proximity, immediacy, and expectation (PIE). Those who recovered were released, while those afflicted with long-term post-traumatic symptoms found it very difficult to gain recognition as wounded veterans. Physicians and psychiatrists generally regarded the issue as one of the army's lowest priorities, a kind of necessary evil, and neither documented their experiences nor preserved the limited knowledge gained in treating trauma sufferers during the war. Military authorities similarly washed their hands of the matter when the war ended (Bleich 2000). Amichai Levy notes that in the entire body of official military medical literature of the period, the problem of CSR goes entirely unmentioned, with the exception of three articles that appeared in *Harefuah* (Medicine) in 1948–1949 (Levy et al. 1989). These articles, for their part, reflect the prevailing Israeli attitudes of the time rather than the authors' medical knowledge. The three authors, all experienced physicians, ascribed to those afflicted with CSR the intention to evade their duties or ideological weakness. They maintained that psychological reactions occurred infrequently among IDF soldiers because of their love of the homeland and their willingness to fight on its behalf. Such attitudes resemble the widely accepted notion from WWI that patriotism could render the soul immune to injury, and that soldiers could cope with any horror so long as they remained faithful to their people. The authors chose to interpret the data available to them in the spirit of these once-common beliefs.

One of the authors, Dr. Kulmus, a former German army physician who had managed a military hospital during WWI, attributes CSR to "a conscious or unconscious desire to evade military service," or in some cases "a lust for compensation." Despite acknowledging that "unstinting sacrifice brings with it psychological shocks of the greatest severity," and despite calling for the establishment of a special department to care for such patients, whose numbers he expected to be great, he adhered to the ideas that had been current among German military physicians during WWI, viewing CSR as a "disease of the will" and a manifestation of the "hysterical mechanism." Echoing opinions of these German physicians, he proposed a brief period of treatment of just a few days' duration, followed by a discharge of the patient from the army. "The expeditious removal of these elements," he explained, "prevents complications and exorbitant expenditure, and no compensation need be paid" (Kulmus 1949).

The second article on war trauma published in this period evinces both admiration of the young soldiers of the Hebrew state and adherence to once-prevalent beliefs in the power of ideology to prevent CSR. The author, Dr. Wolman, a neurologist and psychiatrist, maintained that only a small percentage of Soviet soldiers had suffered psychological injuries during the Nazi invasion of Russia. Though he offered no proof, the author attributed this psychological fortitude to patriotism: "The Soviet soldier's astonishing psychological health should unquestionably be credited to his deep love of his homeland." He was similarly admiring of Israeli soldiers:

> The Hebrew soldier, his moral and ideological level, are, without a doubt, exceedingly high. The Hebrew youth loves his homeland deeply, and his desire and guiding principle are to loyally serve his people and his country.

> Every young man in Israel is willing at all times to take his place in the line of defense. From their earliest childhood, they are reared in a climate of pioneering and national values, and, on reaching maturity, the fire of the nation's exalted ideals burns in their hearts.
>
> (Wolman 1948, p. 40)

He assumed that the acute existential conflict that characterizes CSR—between the instinctive desire to flee an immediate threat to one's life and the imperative to remain and to keep fighting—had little chance of developing among Israeli soldiers:

> For us, there is no choice. Our war is for the very physical survival of the Yishuv and of every single Jew in the Yishuv. The urge to self-defense tells us: Fight, fight until victory is won. Flee the warfront? To where? Is there any place that is safe for a Jew except his land, which he will defend with all his might?
>
> (Wolman 1948, p. 40)

The common negative image of the CSR sufferer is represented in its crudest form in the third article, by Dr. Lipman Heilperin, future head of the neurology department at Hadassah Hospital in Jerusalem and author of the Hebrew Physician's Oath. In this article, he identifies CSR with a lack of desire to fight, a characteristic of "weaklings" and those drafted "by default" through the general mobilization enacted during the second stage of the war. These soldiers had families and businesses, and "a fair number of them were psychically unprepared for action" (Heilperin 1949, p. 12).

These three articles reflect unwillingness on the part of the physicians to apply existing knowledge of the objective causes of CSR to soldiers in Israel's War of Independence. Heilperin exhibited a particularly disparaging view of soldiers drawn from the population of recently arrived Holocaust survivors. Rather than bringing diagnostic skills to bear on their responses to combat, Heilperin merely gave expression to the view, commonly held at the time, that the new immigrants made inferior soldiers, hampered by the same weakness and conformity that let the Jews of Europe go to their deaths "like lambs to the slaughter." Yet his data clearly point to a reactivation of post-traumatic reaction, in which the residual effects of a prior traumatic incident become intensified upon exposure to similar events in the present (Solomon et al. 1987). Heilperin's analysis of the Holocaust-survivor soldiers, which ignored existing knowledge on the topic and placed the responsibility for a psychological injury on the shoulders of the victim rather than on the events that caused it, is reminiscent of the way American psychiatrists disregarded the Holocaust experience and attributed survivors' disorders to innate personality flaws, as described in the previous chapter.

Heilperin's view reflects the larger encounter between the Yishuv and the Holocaust survivors, one marked by opposing expectations: the encounter between the "new Jews" of pre-state Israel and the survivors of the Holocaust occurred in summer 1945, with the arrival of the first emissaries of the Yishuv to the Displaced Persons (DP) camps in Germany, Austria, and Italy. After Israel's declaration of independence in May 1948, Holocaust survivors began arriving in large numbers, even as war raged. By the end of 1949, almost 200,000 survivors had settled in Israel, and relations between Yishuv society mobilized for war and these new immigrants were infused with high expectations and stereotypical beliefs.[6] On the one hand, there existed a commonly held view among the Jewish population of Palestine that a lengthy period of socialization would be necessary for the newly arriving survivors to become partners in the Zionist enterprise. But prevailing fears of defeat in the imminent war prompted Yishuv representatives to expect that the survivors immediately join the struggle for statehood (Keynan 1996). These expectations were, in fact, exceeded when 7,800 survivors from German DP camps alone enlisted in the IDF while still in the camps, more than double the number the Yishuv's representatives had hoped for (Keynan 1996). As the battles raged, Holocaust survivors were assigned to combat units even before they had learned Hebrew, sometimes without appropriate military training. Their Holocaust background, together with the preparation and the language gap, reinforced the stereotype of the refugee soldiers as weak and unable to fight, though it had little basis in reality (Yablonka 2006). So prevalent was this image that the prominence of Holocaust survivors among the IDF soldiers in the well-known battle of Latrun served in Israeli public consciousness—erroneously but conveniently—as an explanation for Israel's defeat in that battle (Shapira 1994). Many within the Yishuv regarded the War of Independence as the war of Israeli youth, while the refugee soldiers, conscripted within the framework of GAHAL (*Giyus Hutz-La'aretz*, Overseas Recruits), were considered to be minor players who were given the "privilege" of joining the war effort (and, by extension, Yishuv society), and the opportunity to avenge the indignity of the Holocaust. The survivors who joined in the war, unless belonging in their past to the Ghetto fighters or the partisans, seemed incapable of meeting the high standards of IDF soldiers, a belief that reinforced and was reinforced by the myth of *sabra* insusceptibility to combat stress. Attributing a "wimpish" image to Holocaust survivors was easy, and aligned with existing perceptions of the difference between the new immigrants and the *sabras*, and of the need of the survivors to adapt to the Zionist high demands of the individual. The same spirit, labeling any weakness as disgrace, enabled the denial of CSR among Israeli soldiers as a whole. This attitude created a similar undermining by IDF *sabras* of their fellow soldiers—both CSR casualties and Holocaust survivors.

The three articles discussed earlier also illustrate how Israeli clinicians during the War of Independence, like their counterparts during the two world wars, subjugated their professional duties to national imperatives. These imperatives and the need to galvanize a cohesive fighting collective shaped the desired traits of an ideal "Israeliness" (Bar-On et al. n.d.; Keynan 1998). Failure to meet these standards excluded the individual from the collective and labeled him or her a coward. Soldiers should display resilience in all situations—as if being afflicted with CSR were a matter of choice—while new immigrants and Holocaust survivors seeking to prove their "Israeliness" should abandon their "exilic" habits and conform to the imperatives of their new identity.

These articles highlight the illusive boundaries between individual and collective trauma in Israeli conceptions. The temporal proximity between Israel's founding and the Holocaust accentuated the sense of the country's role as the solution to the Jewish people's traumatic past. The newly free homeland and its army would liberate the Jewish people from their status as eternal victims and replace the experience of oppression with empowerment. A collective ethos that eclipsed individual experience was necessary to inculcate a sense of absolute sacrifice and fearlessness in soldiers, particularly in so fateful a war as the War of Independence. Emerging in pre-state Israel in the early twentieth century, and aggravated by the Holocaust, the "no choice" narrative—a widely held belief that the Jews in Israel were forced to be strong and always fight to protect their lives, and that this constant existential struggle is the fate of the Jews—reached its peak during the War of Independence, superseding all individual hardship. Amid this tension between collective and individual hardship, priority was always given to the former, and the greater the sense of collective danger, the stronger the tendency to disregard personal trauma. So many emotional resources were spent to alleviate the historical burden of national trauma and bolster the independent Jewish state that almost none remained to address the war's impact on the individual psyche.

It is no coincidence that Dr. Wolman also attributed the personal "immunity" to CSR of every soldier at the front to the collective determination of a society convinced that it was fighting for its survival. As he saw it, one moved by love of his or her homeland and concern for her people is necessarily immune to combat stress. Such attitudes made any soldier who experienced combat stress suspect and unpatriotic: if love of the homeland is a prophylactic, then those afflicted with combat stress clearly lack devotion. It takes reasoning of this kind, during a period of this kind, to explain the incident in which soldiers from the Palmach elite Brigade Harel gloated over the suffering of 15 traumatized fellow soldiers, who hid under a convalescent home in Kibbutz Kiryat Anavim (near Jerusalem) rather than participate in the fighting when the building was attacked (Bar-On et al. n.d.).

Amichai Levy (Levy et al. 1989) views this attitude as one of the reasons why, even after the War of Independence, Israel did not establish a system for treating or studying combat reactions, and, in fact, the IDF dismantled its few mental health centers. The establishment of such a system might have been interpreted as anticipation of future combat trauma, which in turn might have cast doubt on the motivation and resilience of Israeli soldiers. Dan Bar-On et al. (n.d.) suggest an additional reason: there was no need to preserve or understand those traumatic experiences amassed during the war because it was assumed that such responses would disappear without a trace once the new immigrants had become fully subsumed within the *sabra* "melting pot" (Bar-On et al. n.d.). To legitimize CSR would threaten the myth of the *sabra* itself and, more importantly, blur the boundaries that demarcated for the collective what was permitted and what was forbidden. It was easier—and essential to the preservation of national myths—to see CSR as an aberrant phenomenon, and those afflicted with it as deserters, cowards, or weaklings. It is interesting to note that although the Palmach was the bastion of "Israeliness" within the IDF, the Holocaust survivors drafted into it integrated more successfully than did the survivors who joined other units. Hannah Yablonka attributes this to the communal support provided by the Palmach, a relatively small, closed group (Yablonka 1999). But their successful absorption can also be ascribed to the influence of the aforementioned myths. Those who joined the elite unit found in them a clear and open path into the narrative of heroism and into "Israeliness."

Israeli attitudes toward the Holocaust survivors during and after the War of Independence were marked by contradiction rooted in an ambivalent view of the Holocaust as a source of both weakness and strength: precisely because it brought the Jewish people as a whole to the brink of destruction, this unprecedented catastrophe continues to fuel the nation's resolve to prevent any future trauma—"never again." Vamik Volkan uses the term "living monument" to describe the trauma victims who represent a collective history of victimhood and a shared national or ethnic identity (Volkan 1990). In Israel, the term is sometimes used to describe the bereaved families of the IDF soldiers, but it can just as readily be applied to the Holocaust survivors (Witztum & Malkinson 1993).[7] One feature of the "living monument" is its straddling of two worlds: the survivors are honored in the sphere of shared identity, their suffering is appropriated as part of the collective experience, yet they also suffer alone in a nightmare of personal pain. This duality, not unique to Israel, characterizes survivors of trauma who, for their nation, symbolize both the existential threat and the possibility of rebirth. Because recognition of personal trauma threatens to sap the broader potential for heroism, we often see this same duality at work in the states' treatment of soldiers returning from war. Although the nation glorifies the warriors and the war from which they have returned, the soldiers themselves frequently remain alone with their nightmares and memories and, in some cases, these post-traumatic experiences accompany them throughout their lives.

When the War of Independence ended (1949), IDF leaderships dismantled the small military mental health system. Seven years later, during the Sinai War, 5% of the wounded apparently suffered from CSR (Levy et al. 1990), though the army continued to ignore the phenomenon, and the public was left with the impression that no combat-related trauma had been suffered during this war. This lack of preparation for and dismissal of combat stress continued to characterize the Israeli military establishment both before and during the Six-Day War in 1967. Psychiatrists and mental health officers, who, by this point, recognized the phenomenon's existence, tried to establish rules and treatment methodologies, but the IDF maintained the official position that commitment inoculated soldiers against trauma (Levy et al. 1990).

The speed of Israel's victory in the Six-Day War often obscures the tense period that preceded its outbreak. The country prepared itself for heavy casualties, and a sense of immediate existential threat took hold of the Israeli public. The danger was experienced as real and tangible and, for many, was emotionally linked to the

Holocaust because of awareness awakened a few years earlier by the Eichmann trial. A perusal of the well-known collection of interviews *The Seventh Day: Soldiers' Talk about the Six-Day War* highlights the impression that these feelings had intensified among the soldiers, who viewed the war as a life-or-death event: "We were not fighting for the territory itself, we were fighting for our lives" (Shapira 1968, p. 160).[8] During this period the "no choice" narrative and a sense of the Jews' tragic destiny amid "never-ending wars" became even more deeply entrenched (Shapira 1968). *Sabra* soldiers who had been born after the Holocaust and who, up to this point, had often related to the memory of that period with indifference now became aware of it: "Suddenly everyone starts talking about Munich, about the Holocaust, and about the forsaken Jewish people . . ." (Shapira 1968, p. 7).

After the war, deep apprehension gave way to the euphoria of victory, and the *sabra* myth soared to new heights. The media broadcasts and print publications that prior to and during the war had been devoted to raising morale now heaped praise upon what had come to be perceived as the greatest army in the world. The festive national mood eclipsed the mourning for the loss of 800 dead and concern for the pain of 2,600 wounded Israeli soldiers.[9] The families of the casualties, according to Professor Ephraim Urbach, whose own son was killed in combat shortly after the war,[10] felt "isolated in their sorrow and grief, as the entire land rang with the joy of victory" (quoted in Shamir 1976, p. 14). Only a year after the war, when the bodies of the dead soldiers were being transferred for permanent interment in military cemeteries, did the newspapers devote significant space to articles memorializing their sacrifice. Despite the central place of bereavement in the national ethos, the bereaved individual remained alone, in the shadows of the myth of heroism.

A huge chasm exists between the state's treatment of bereaved families and, to a lesser degree, physically wounded soldiers and the state's treatment of CSR sufferers. The nation exalts the former while dismissing, even belittling, the latter. Yet the two attitudes are connected. The myth of heroism destines the bereaved and physically wounded to serve as a kind of a "living monument," symbolizing the glory of war and victory, while assigning them the duty of bearing their grief alone, in silence. The same myth condemns the CSR casualties to exclusion from the glory of the warrior altogether, portraying them as a burden on the nation.

When it seemed as though Israel might be obliterated from the map, the nation reverted to the former pre-state model of general mobilization, a universal spirit of self-sacrifice, and the denial of the very idea of psychological injury. Victory having been attained, adoration was showered upon the soldiers who, in the space of six days, had managed to transform a state on the brink of annihilation into a regional power. Such adoration left no room for a soldier's traumatic war experience.

Professor Eliezer Witztum, then a teenager who served as a volunteer stretcher-bearer in an Afula[11] hospital during the Six-Day War, recounts a specific incident from the war that illustrates both the depth of denial that prevailed at the end of Israel's second decade of existence and how CSR sufferers were once again abandoned by the IDF medical establishment. In an interview with *Yedioth Ahronoth* (a leading Israeli newspaper) reporter Yigal Sarna, he relates his astonishment at the sight of a tank crewman in scorched clothes, who had come straight from the battle at Emek Dotan:

> The soldier looked battle-shocked. Physical examination revealed no physical injury. The senior surgeon went up to him, slapped him hard on the face. "Pretender," he yelled, "you're taking the place of a real casualty," and shoved him off the bed and out of the emergency room. The stunned soldier wasn't even able to talk and, to this day, I can't forget his eyes.
>
> (Sarna 1990)

End of the Era of Denial: The Yom Kippur War (1973)

The Yom Kippur War, a major collective trauma, has become seared into Israeli national memory, and much has been written about the war's political, military, and social repercussions (Shemesh & Drori 2008). One outcome of the war was the official recognition of combat reactions for the first time in the country's history. The IDF instituted comprehensive reforms, support treatment, research, and a range of services for trauma sufferers. These reforms helped legitimize the plight of the syndrome's victims and foster greater awareness of CSR within the military establishment.

Most scholars attribute the timing of the recognition of CSR in Israel to the collective trauma of the Yom Kippur War, as the myth of the invincible Israeli soldier was shattered and the vast number of soldiers traumatized in the war made continued denial impossible (Bleich 2000; Levy et al. 1990 (2)). These explanations, though correct in and of themselves, do not adequately account for the realignment of the deeply entrenched societal attitudes that placed national existential danger above individual suffering. The sense of threat experienced by Israel during the Yom Kippur War ought to have led to a reactivation of the earlier modes of denial and dismissal in the face of any sign of weakness on the part of those charged with defending the nation. Indeed, a portion of the Israeli public continued to deny the relevance of individual suffering at a time of collective danger. As a soldier from Kfar Etzion[12] remarked, illustrating widespread efforts directed at collective self-scrutiny after the war, "A person going into battle has to think the big thoughts, not the small ones. [. . .] If the Jewish people needs this struggle, who am I, and what is my life worth?" (quoted in Feige 2008, p. 360).

The change in attitude toward CSR thus requires another explanation. The Yom Kippur War triggered profound changes in the Israeli public's view of the soldier's experience and the way that experience was represented. Absent from Israel's collective memory in the immediate aftermath of the Yom Kippur War were the symbols of heroism that had predominated in the past, despite the many instances of personal heroism (Witztum & Malkinson 1993). The rhetoric of war changed, and heroic national myths gave way to emphasis on the price that war exacts on the individual. This new narrative grew out of the spontaneous protest movements that were spearheaded by IDF reservists and spread to the general public. The reservists' protest sought to dispel the myths that shrouded the mistakes and miscalculations responsible for Israel's unpreparedness for the war, and to bring to light the pain of those ordinary soldiers who suffered for the ineptitude and arrogance of the military and political leadership. The alarmingly high death toll was thus attributed to a failure of leadership, while only the personal heroism exhibited by the soldiers was recognized as having saved the country from annihilation. The dreadful war was regarded by the Israeli public as an instance of the sins of the fathers being visited upon the sons: the younger generation paid the price for the older generation's complacency.

The changing rhetoric of the soldier's experience—from heroism to suffering—enabled the Israeli public and the IDF to cease denying the existence of combat reactions (Feige 2008). This change also shifted the discourse on the individual's duty of self-sacrifice for the good of the state to a discourse on reciprocity between the state and those it sends into battle.

One could say that the Israeli public as a whole suffered from collective CSR in the wake of the Yom Kippur War, a reaction born of the sense of immediate existential danger, the public's loss of faith in its leadership, and the shattering of the collective illusion of safety that had prevailed since the euphoric victory of the Six-Day War.[13] The impact of the trauma was manifested in anger and fear. Anger shaped the public's memory of the war as a preventable episode and as punishment for the smugness of the Israeli leadership. Fear intensified the public's sense of having to reconcile itself to an intractable state of living under perpetual threat. While the war reinforced the narrative of Israel's need to defend itself resolutely and continuously, it also cultivated a new narrative, according to which the war had been unnecessary, or at least its scope could have been reduced, and the harm to soldiers minimized had Israel's military and civilian leaders conducted themselves more responsibly.

Both narratives encompassed a growing awareness of the price paid by soldiers, and thereby highlighted the tension between individual and collective trauma, a tension that had previously been suppressed by national mythology. Many of the parents of the soldiers who fought in the Yom Kippur War had themselves fought in 1948. Seeing the suffering reflected in the eyes of their children as they returned from a war that had come to be publicly regarded as a blunder, many members of the Palmach generation questioned the old myths, which now began to seem hollow.[14] This was the emotional foundation of the paradigm change concerning CSR, and it had a hand in shaping the discussion of reciprocity and the state's obligation toward its soldiers. The chain of command in the IDF and the Ministry of Defense began to implement some of the psychological knowledge that they had previously rejected. In doing so, they fell in step with changes taking place around the world, culminating in 1980, when the American Psychiatric Association's *Diagnostic and Statistical Manual of Mental Disorders* recognized combat and post-traumatic reactions as syndromes caused by traumatic events, unrelated to any preexisting or congenital disorders.[15]

The IDF's initial estimate of 700 CSR casualties in the Yom Kippur War, which at first seemed high, was actually much lower than the true figure. When the

Medical Corps collected data on war wounded not diagnosed during the war, the researchers concluded that more than 2,000 soldiers (30% of all war wounded) suffered from deep psychological scars (Sarna 1990).[16] Most of the wounded had received insufficient or inappropriate treatment by the IDF, which had failed to apply Salmon's proximity and immediacy principles.[17] Many other cases of CSR and PTSD went unidentified and entirely untreated, which lowered the sufferers' chances of recovery. Many of the 301 Israeli prisoners of war, for example, suffered from PTSD and experienced exceptionally severe difficulties adjusting after their release. Returning POWs were accorded a half-hearted welcome, described by many of them as a trauma in and of itself. They were given no appropriate treatment until 1998, when, in response to the efforts of the organization Erim Balayla ("Awake at Night"), the Ministry of Defense finally offered them treatment and psychological aid.[18] Nevertheless, the legitimacy of war-related psychological injury had been established, and an array of services was now being provided by the IDF Medical Corps, both in times of emergency and in times of peace. The IDF began formulating therapeutic methods and proved increasingly capable of coping with soldiers' psychological injuries. The IDF integrated psychiatrists and therapists into various combat units, created an infrastructure for CSR research, and made efforts to raise awareness about combat stress among soldiers and commanders and teach preventive methods (Shklar 1990).

Notes

1. Uzi Narkiss in an interview with Boaz Lev Tov, the Yitzhak Rabin Center for Israel Studies, quoted in Bar-On et al. (n.d.). Narkiss (1925–1997) was an Israeli general, who fought in Israeli war of independence (1948) and in the Six-Day War (1967).
2. Although attempts have been made by some scholars to refute the Israeli belief of "the few against many," such critiques do not take into account the fact that the Yishuv (the Jewish community in pre-state Israel) devoted all of its resources, human and economic, to the war effort, and that these resources came close to being exhausted. Thus, the question of whether in a given battle the IDF had more or fewer weapons or soldiers is irrelevant and fails to reflect the overall reality of the war.
3. Strong farmer and warrior. See Keynan (1990, 1996).
4. See Moshe Tabenkin's poem "Eulogy": "Our youth was lofty as the cliffs of the Gilboa Mountains, soaring eagle-like, brave and daring, ascending higher and higher until his last moments before the foe." Cited in Raizen (1995).
5. Bereaved father Eliezer Kalir, in a poem published in *Davar HaShavua*, 9 May 1951. See also Keynan (2000).
6. From among 340,000 new immigrants who arrived between 15 May 1948 and the end of 1949 (Central Bureau of Statistics [CBS] 2012). On the tensions between the survivors and veteran Israelis, see Keynan (1996); Yablonka (1999).
7. Witztum and Malkinson emphasize, in this context, the bereaved families of the War of Independence—families that, in their view, constitute a "living monument" to those who fell in that war—young men who symbolized the revival of the nation that had lost 6 million of its people.
8. An English edition, edited by Henry Near, is also available.
9. Casualty figures from Yariv (1985).
10. www.izkor.gov.il/HalalKorot.aspx?id=90083.
11. A small city in the north district of Israel in the middle of the Yizrael Valley, very near to the pre-1967 Jordanian border.

12. Kfar Etzion is a small religious kibbutz near Jerusalem, which was first established in 1927. In 1948, the Arab Legion conquered it, massacred 157 of its Jewish inhabitants, and destroyed it. It then remained under Jordanian rule until 1967, when it was reestablished.
13. The term "illusion of safety" is used here in its meaning of defense against extreme fear in wartime. See the relevant discussion in Chapter 1.
14. On reflections of this deep change in societal beliefs regarding war, CSR, and heroism, see Arbel (2008); Levin (2000).
15. As noted in note 6 of the introduction, in 1980 PTSD was included in the DSM for the first time as a separate syndrome related to combat stress reaction.
16. Sarna quotes Shabtai Noy: "Even today, veterans of the Yom Kippur War are coming to the CSR unit after years of suffering untreated." See also Levy interview, 2009. Also Gabi Weissman, then the IDF's chief mental health officer, submitted a report on the topic to the chief medical officer after the war, and even appealed to the Agranat Commission to investigate the mental health system's wartime performance. The Agranat Commission was a national commission of inquiry set up to investigate the failure of the IDF to prepare for the Yom Kippur War (1973).
17. See Chapter 2.
18. On the returning POWs see Neria et al. (2000). On the relationship between the parents of the POWs and the state, see Hasson-Rochlin (2006). Although it is beyond the purview of this book, it should be noted that the status of traumatized POWs is more complex than that of those afflicted with PTSD or CSR under other conditions. That said, both constitute instances of post-traumatic stress, and relevant to both is the reciprocal relationship between the soldiers and the system that sent them on their trauma-inducing missions.

References

Almog, O. 1998, *The Sabra: a Portrait*, Am Oved, Tel Aviv. (Hebrew)

Arbel, S. (director) (2008). *Shurot Shurot*. Amutat Ohalei Palmach, Tel Aviv.

Bar-On, D., Bar, L., & Rom, A. (n.d.) *The Social Function of the Non-Reporting of Combat Stress Reaction during the 1948 War*, unpublished manuscript. (Hebrew)

Bleich, A. 2000, 'Military Psychiatry in Israel: a 50-Year Perspective', *Harefuah*, vol. 138, no. 9, pp. 728–733.

CBS, *Statistical Abstract of Israel 2012*. Available from www.cbs.gov.il [June 18 2013].

Feige, M. 2008, 'The Yom Kippur War in Israeli Memory: Rupture with the Past Versus Continuity' in *National Trauma: the Yom Kippur War: a Retrospective of Thirty Years and Another War*, eds. M. Shemesh & Z. Drori, Ben-Gurion Institute and Ben-Gurion University, Sde Boker, pp. 351–366.

Hasson-Rochlin, Y. 2006, *Parenthood to Soldiers in Israel as a Political Resource*, master's degree thesis, Open University.

Heilperin, L. 1949, 'Neuropsychiatric Observations in the Jerusalem War', *Harefuah*, vol. 36, no., 1, pp. 11–13. (Hebrew)

Keynan, I. 1990, 'Between Hope and Fear: the Image of the She'erit HaPleita in the Eyes of the Jewish Emissaries from Palestine to the Displaced Persons Camps in Germany, 1945' in *Ha'apala, Studies in the History of Illegal Immigrants*, ed. A. Shapira, Am Oved, Tel Aviv, pp. 211–229.

Keynan, I. 1996, *The Hunger Has Not Abated: the Surviving Remnants of the Holocaust and the Israeli Pre-State Emissaries, 1945–1948*, Am Oved Press, Tel Aviv. (Hebrew)

Keynan, I. 1998, *The Lust for Heroism and the Disgrace of Weakness: Holocaust Survivors and Combat Stress Reaction Sufferers in the War of Independence*, [Lecture delivered at the Conference Marking 50 Years of Statehood, the Historical Society], April. (Hebrew)

Keynan, I. 2000, 'The Memory of Bereavement as a Legacy Entrusted to Israel's Youth' in *For Yom HaZikaron* [Remembrance Day], Ministry of Defense, Department of Families and Remembrance, Tel Aviv.

Kulmus, A. 1949, 'On War Neurosis', *Harefuah*, vol. 36, no. 3–4, pp. 43–44. (Hebrew)

Levin, H. 2000, 'Queen of the Bathtub' in *What Does the Bird Care: Hanoch Levin's Collected Writings*, Hakibbutz Hameuchad and Sifrei, Tel Aviv.

Levy, A., Witztum, E., Granek, M., & Kotler, M. 1989, 'Combat Reactions in Israel's Wars, 1948–1973, Part 1: General Background and History, Methodology and a Review of the Literature of the Period', *Sichot*, vol. 4, no. 1, pp. 60–70. (Hebrew)

Levy, A., Witztum, E., Granek, M., & Kotler, M. 1990, 'Combat Reactions in Israel's Wars, 1948–1973, Part 4: the Six-Day War, 1967', *Sichot*, vol. 4, no. 3, pp. 217–221. (Hebrew)

Levy, A., Witztum, E., Granek, M., & Kotler, M. 1990 (2), 'The Treatment of Combat Reactions in the IDF, 1948–1973', *Harefuah*, vol. 32, pp. 49–53. (Hebrew)

Neria, Y., Solomon, Z., Dekel, R., & Ginzburg, K. 2000, 'Returning Yom Kippur War POWs: Predictors of Adjustment Problems and Therapeutic/Rehabilitative Issues', *Society and Welfare* [*Hevra URevaha*], vol. 20, no. 2, pp. 159–174. (Hebrew)

Raizen, E. 1995, *No Rattling of Sabers, an Anthology of Israeli War Poetry*, University of Texas Press, Austin.

Sarna, Y. 1990, 'The Battle Shock Blunder', *Yedioth Ahronoth*, 28 November. (Hebrew)

Shamir, I. (ed.) 1976, *Commemoration and Its Meaning: Issues in the Commemoration of Fallen IDF Soldiers*, Ministry of Defense, Rehabilitation Division, Tel Aviv.

Shapira, A. (ed.) 1968, *The Seventh Day: Soldiers' Talk about the Six-Day War*; recorded and edited by a group of young kibbutz members. (Hebrew)

Shapira, A. 1994, 'Historiography and Memory: Latrun, 1948', *Alpayim (2000), a Multidisciplinary Publication for Contemporary Thought and Literature*, no. 10, pp. 9–41. (Hebrew)

Shemesh, M., & Drori, Z. (eds.) (2008), *National Trauma: the Yom Kippur War: a Retrospective of Thirty Years and Another War*, Ben-Gurion Institute and Ben-Gurion University, Sde Boker.

Shklar, R. 1990, 'Mental Health in Uniform—the Development of the IDF's Mental Health System', *Bit'on Hel HaRefuah* [*I.D.F. Medical Corps Bulletin*], vol. 32, pp. 5–7.

Sivan, E. 1991, *The 1948 Generation: Myth, Portrait and Memory*, Ma'arachot, Tel Aviv. (Hebrew)

Solomon, Z., Garb, R., Bleich, A., & Grupper, D. 1987, 'Reactivation of Combat Stress among Israeli Soldiers in the Lebanon War', *Sichot*, vol. 2, no. 1, pp. 31–36. (Hebrew)

Volkan, V. D. 1990, 'Living Status and Political Decision-Making', *Mind and Human Interaction*, vol. 2, no. 2, pp. 46–50.

Witztum, E., & Malkinson, R. 1993, 'Bereavement and Memorialization: the Two Faces of the National Myth' in *Loss and Bereavement in Jewish Society in Israel*, eds. E. Witztum & R. Malkinson, Kanah and the Ministry of Defense, Tel Aviv, pp. 231–258. (Hebrew)

Wolman, B. 1948, 'Some Problems of Psychic Hygiene and Military Psychiatry', *Harefuah*, vol. 35, no. 5–6, pp. 39–41. (Hebrew)

Yablonka, H. 1999, *Survivors of the Holocaust: Israel after the War*, New York University Press, New York.

Yablonka, H. 2006, 'Holocaust Survivors in the Israeli Army during the 1948 War: Documents and Memory', *Israel Affairs*, vol. 12, no. 3, pp. 462–483.

Yablonka, H. (n.d.), *The Holocaust Survivors in the War of Independence*. Available from www.yadvashem.org/yv/he/exhibitions/survivors/book/yablunka.pdf [June 16, 2013].

Yariv, A. 1985, 'War of Choice and War of No-Choice' in *War by Choice: Essays*, ed. A. Yariv, Hakibbutz Hameuchad, Tel Aviv, pp. 9–30, Kav Adom series.

4 "The Helicopter Isn't Coming"[1]

The Wounded and the System

The IDF's Combat Stress Reaction Unit

Four years after the Yom Kippur War, the Israeli Defense Forces (IDF) treatment facility for CSR conducted its first drill to identify and treat CSR casualties during combat. A few years later, the Disabled Rehabilitation Division at the Ministry of Defense (RDMD) founded a military unit to study and treat war trauma, which has remained an active presence in the field ever since (Shklar 1990; Solomon 1993).[2] The unit established standards and methods for the immediate treatment of soldiers at the front, rather than only after their evacuation from the battlefield, as well as for those suffering from delayed-onset or continuous post-traumatic reactions after discharge from the IDF.[3] Since its founding, the unit has treated over 2,000 CSR casualties, most of them veterans of the 1973 Yom Kippur War and the 1982 First Lebanon War. The unit also constantly invests in research and in improvement of treatment methods. This bore fruit during the Second Lebanon War in 2006, when sophisticated diagnostic tools for the immediate identification of CSR casualties were implemented with great success.

The State of Israel currently recognizes CSR and PTSD as "legitimate" injuries that confer entitlement to psychological support and constitute grounds for disability claims. The distinction between CSR and PTSD and other non-security-related disorders suffered by soldiers (e.g., psychosis, schizophrenia) has been legislatively addressed by the Israeli Parliament (Knesset) (*The Disability Law* 2000). Accordingly, security-related PTSD is distinguished from other psychological disorders in the defense establishment's disability rating schedule.[4] These measures mark an important policy shift from the long-standing official denial of psychological trauma and the tendency to view it as a disease or preexisting mental disorder, rather than a war injury. However, this legislation and the related disability rating remain controversial, and have been opposed to on the grounds of being excessively generous, populist gestures.[5]

Significant progress has also been made in the attitudes of IDF officers toward CSR. A 1989 study found that officers generally accepted CSR among low-ranking soldiers, although participants in the study expressed reservations about officers afflicted with CSR, believing that they should "take responsibility" for their recovery (Inbar et al. 1989). Although this perspective reflected a limited understanding of CSR and persistence of the stigma attributed to individuals with CSR, the sympathetic view of the officers toward traumatized enlisted soldiers reflected a real change. Another sign of the change in attitudes within the IDF was seen in 1995. A study of that year found that mental health officers in the military no longer attributed CSR to personality flaws, cowardice, or a desire to shirk one's duties, but rather to external circumstances, such as harsh battle conditions, food and sleep deprivation, or, sometimes, a lack of support from fellow soldiers or commanding officers (Shalom et al. 1995). According to the researchers, this change in attitude among mental health officers reflected new IDF training and policy that defined CSR as a normal, transitional crisis caused by exposure to combat stress (ibid.).

In a way, the Israeli CSR Unit has been doing what the DSM-5 Task Force expects the American army to do (in response to the army's request to change the syndrome's name from disorder to injury [American Psychological Association 2013]): change the atmosphere within the army and reduce social barriers to veterans in asking for help. The change can be partly attributed to the activities of the CSR Unit, which has worked since its establishment to raise awareness about combat trauma within the army, and has devoted efforts to what the unit terms "primary prevention," offering workshops and lectures and disseminating literature on trauma to officers. The unit works closely with IDF mental health professionals, trains personnel for the immediate treatment of trauma ("secondary prevention"), and offers further care to those who were treated on the battlefield but have not yet recovered ("tertiary prevention"). For trauma injuries that were not identified at the time they occurred, wounded servicemen are eligible for treatment by the CSR Unit at any point in time, even years after discharge.[6]

Although the current benefit package, comprising psychological support, financial benefits, and treatment, appears to signal a significant improvement in defense establishment attitudes toward soldiers afflicted with CSR and PTSD, we are still a long way from optimal treatment procedures or a complete erasure of the stigma of CSR, as I show ahead. Moreover, recent policy decisions—adopted by the Disabled Rehabilitation Division at the Ministry of Defense (RDMD)—that restrict the treatment period to 12–18 months endanger patient recovery,[7] especially in some cases where treatment may be prematurely suspended due to increasingly stringent Defense Ministry criteria.

The Wounded and the Defense Establishment: The Helicopter Isn't Coming for Us

Every soldier who has been mentally or physically wounded may claim benefits and/or medical assistance from the Ministry of Defense. The military system is responsible for providing treatment to soldiers as long as they are in active service, and the RDMD is responsible for veterans, including reserve soldiers. Typically, the physically wounded are immediately released from service, and then may claim benefits and medical care from the RDMD. Due to the diagnostic challenges of PTSD, and since symptoms are often delayed, a soldier may still be in active service when he or she seeks psychological support and treatment. As a result, active service members are treated by the CSR Unit.

Similar to the US procedure, the claims process for all wounded soldiers begins with an application for benefits and medical care directed to the RDMD. The RDMD collects all necessary details, reviews the causal connection between the claimant's disability and military service, refers the applicant to a medical committee (whose members are physicians and psychiatrists) that issues a medical opinion, and ultimately decides whether to recognize the claimant as a disabled IDF veteran. Based on the medical committee's determination of the claimant's disability (expressed as a disability percentage), the RDMD decides on the range of services and benefits to award him or her. Naturally, the more severe the injury, the more dependent the claimant is on the benefit system.

In the US, soldiers who are still in service obtain psychological support from the Department of Defense (DOD), while wounded veterans are cared for by the Department of Veterans Affairs (VA), a government agency that provides a wide range of welfare and health services to veterans. Wounded soldiers are eligible for mental and physical treatment and benefits. Claims are filed with the Veterans Benefits Administration (VBA) at the VA, which checks eligibility (Worthen & Moering 2011), and conducts C&P (compensation and pension) reviews to decide whether a direct documented connection exists between the veteran's claim and his or her injury (Moering 2011).

Despite the progress in Israel in the recognition and treatment of CSR and PTSD described earlier, servicemen still paint a picture of isolation, often feeling they have been left to cope and care for themselves.[8] This feeling is very similar to the ambivalent relationship of respect and distrust in the US between veterans and the VA (Finley 2011) and to the feelings of American veterans that no one cares to listen to their pain (CD/IK 2009).[9] In recent Israeli testimonies I collected, documentaries, books written by veterans, investigative reports by journalists, and other sources, soldiers express a variety of criticisms about the system of benefits and care provided by the RDMD. Their complaints range from the medical committees' failure to understand the depth of their needs to much more serious accounts of being treated as a burden on the state budget. Soldiers frequently complain that no proactive efforts are invested to identify those afflicted with psychological trauma, that the medical committees are offensive and humiliating, and that the establishment only grudgingly acknowledges its obligation toward the psychologically wounded, occasionally refusing to extend assistance to claimants with a clear need if their injury does not fit the exact definition of PTSD. Although veterans and soldiers articulate their frustration in many ways, these are effectively summarized in the statement of one traumatized veteran of the Yom Kippur War: "I feel like a wounded soldier on the battlefield, with a helicopter circling overhead that isn't coming down to rescue me" (quoted in Peled 1999).

How can we account for the gap between the progress in formal policy described earlier and the frustration experienced by soldiers? One explanation lies with soldiers' subjective emotional reaction to the realization of the lifelong implications of their injury. Emotional tension naturally develops between an injured party and the system that has sent him or her to war, and now has the obligation to care for him or her. The system often becomes the target of the injured soldier's pain and frustration, rooted in the irresolvable longing to be the person he or she was before the war.[10] The same dynamic has been observed among the physically wounded, but frustration and tension are heightened in the case of the psychologically traumatized, due to the nature of the injury and its symptoms, which include a sense of isolation, abandonment, and distrust.[11]

But this explanation provides only a part of the picture. In fact, the major explanation for the gap between the policy reforms and the persistent experience of frustration of the wounded can be traced to the actual interactions between the Defense Ministry and CSR sufferers.

Caught in the Bureaucratic Web

All soldiers who have suffered a physical or psychological injury during the course of their military service are entitled by law to receive medical care and financial compensation. In the case of trauma casualties, the right to treatment can be exercised through the CSR Unit in the IDF even before eligibility for compensation has been officially determined. However, as noted earlier, the Ministry of Defense places limits on the length of treatment, and the ministry's policies concerning the treatment of traumatized soldiers and the process of applying for benefits are marked by confusion and contradiction. The division of responsibilities between the CSR Unit and the Ministry of Defense can be vague. It is unclear, for example, what happens to a soldier treated by the unit but whose application for benefits is denied by the Defense Ministry. This uncertainty stems from the different criteria of eligibility for treatment applied by the CSR Unit and the RDMD. The army unit treats almost every applicant based on the unit's own diagnosis of his or her psychological situation, regardless of compensation eligibility, while the RDMD provides benefits (including treatment) only to soldiers classified with a disability rating of more than 20%.[12] A special Knesset committee headed by MK (Member of Knesset) Yisrael Hasson in the former administration (henceforth "Hasson Committee") made an attempt to modify this division of treatment. The committee suggested making the CSR Unit responsible for all psychological treatment of trauma casualties, whether they are in service or veterans. If adopted, this would solve two important problems: it would separate treatment from the process of determining eligibility for benefits, thus eliminating the threat of losing eligibility for benefits in the event of a temporary improvement in the claimant's situation; and it would concentrate the responsibility for treatment in a single unit.[13] Unfortunately, the committee's activities were suspended after the administration change following the national January 2013 elections.

In addition, the claim application process is lengthy and frustrating, and often exposes soldiers to the still-prevalent distrust in Israeli society of psychological trauma sufferers in general and benefits claimants in particular. Avi Bleich and Zahava Solomon have shown that only 5% of all applications are examined within a month of submission (Solomon & Bleich 2002). In 48% of claims in their sample, over a year passes from the time a traumatized soldier submits his or her claim until the first medical examination takes place. In 10% of the claims, more than two years elapse before the soldiers undergo a medical exam. While the Ministry of Defense ultimately approved the overwhelming majority of claims reviewed in the study (73% of participants were ultimately classified as disabled, and in only 11% of the cases did the Ministry determine that no connection could be found between the claimant's impairment and his or her military service), the protracted process supports the common feeling among traumatized soldiers that their plight is met with indifference. Bleich and Solomon note elsewhere (Bleich & Solomon 2002) that a 12-month or longer waiting period between symptom onset and disability assessment is reasonable given the need to monitor the syndrome's progress over time and to determine the optimal therapy and rehabilitation program. While the waiting period before the final disability assessment may be justified, there is no justification for such a long waiting period before the first medical examination is conducted, or for the length of the evaluation process as a whole. Indeed, Solomon and Bleich recommend substantially reducing the length of the evaluation process, and find no clinical reason not to do so.

The lengthy evaluation process is just one of the obstacles faced by CSR sufferers. Bleich and Solomon also show that the disability ratings ultimately assigned by the Defense Ministry are frequently too low for adequate compensation and treatment (Solomon & Bleich 2002). Over one-half of the participants in their study (57.4%) were assigned a disability rating of 10% or lower (too low to qualify for assistance or therapy), and only 12% were assigned disability ratings higher than 30%. These ratings, they say, do not adequately reflect the severity of the subjects' conditions as recorded in their study. In another study conducted in conjunction with the Ministry of Defense, designed as a self-assessment of the RDMD's operations, Bleich and Solomon compared the data and disability ratings of all those listed within the Ministry of Defense as psychologically disabled (6,400 IDF veterans) with the findings of three independent evaluation centers to which the Defense Ministry referred a sample of 346 diagnosed veterans, and with World Health Organization data on average disability ratings of PTSD sufferers (Bleich & Solomon 2002). Their findings proved consistent with those of the previous study, supporting the authors' appraisal that the RDMD underevaluates the severity of many claimants' disability. The authors conclude that the large gap between the actual psychological condition of IDF disabled veterans with PTSD and the disability ratings assigned to them demands an in-depth reevaluation of RDMD assessment criteria (Solomon & Bleich 2002).

Bleich and Solomon note that this gap can be explained in part by the theory-based clinical logic used to assign disability ratings, which produces complicated and complex diagnoses according to fixed protocols that often do not meet the actual needs of PTSD sufferers (Bleich & Solomon 2002). This criticism applies also to the DSM's diagnostic criteria for PTSD, which are the basis of the work of the RDMD's medical committees. As elaborated ahead, the symptoms of many traumatized veterans do not always meet the necessary DSM's full criteria for recognition of PTSD, yet often cause distress and functional impairment comparable to that of full-blown PTSD. Depression, anxiety, panic attacks, adjustment problems, and even various forms of addiction are all comorbid with PTSD and can manifest even without the full range of definitive symptoms. This point has been raised in studies and evaluations conducted by experts in Israel and around the world, who all note the limitations of the clinical definition of PTSD, which exclude from recognition and treatment many individuals who experience obvious trauma-related suffering and functional impairments (Skodol et al. 1996; Bleich & Solomon 2002; Tanielian & Jaycox 2008).[14]

In March 2010, Colonel Chaim Knobler, former IDF chief psychiatrist, who, since leaving that post in 2005 has been active in the Association for the Advancement of Combat Stress Reaction Sufferers, addressed the public committee appointed by the Israeli government in 2009, under the leadership of Judge (ret.) Uri Goren (the Goren Committee). The Goren Committee was assigned to study the eligibility criteria for assistance used by the RDMD and the Department of Families and Remembrance, in order to "enhance efficiency and ensure savings within the rehabilitation system."[15] Among other issues, the committee addressed PTSD. Knobler stressed the inadequacies of the diagnostic process:

> In such cases [of functional impairment due to symptoms comorbid with PTSD] . . . there is a tendency on the part of Rehabilitation Division specialists not to diagnose CSR. This means that if all the symptoms necessary for a PTSD diagnosis per the American research manual—not the diagnostic manual but rather the *research* manual—are not present—the disabled person is told: *You have a psychological problem caused during combat, but it isn't CSR, because you don't have PTSD.*[16]

Frustration and disappointment with the systems that diagnose and treat CSR that results in PTSD are not unique to Israel. In Canada, for example, recognition of PTSD and comorbid disabilities takes years, and claims are often rejected due to a similar discrepancy between the diagnostic protocol and claimants' symptoms. Psychologically wounded Canadian veterans have described their return from service as an experience entailing suffering, alienation, or the feeling that the army has thrust them aside "like an object" or "like an old rag" (*Operation Retour* 2005).[17] A major American study conducted by the Rand Corporation in 2008 also revealed widespread lack of access to treatment, and found that one-half of the sufferers from PTSD and depression returning from service in Iraq or Afghanistan did not receive even minimally appropriate treatment. This study and others highlight the logistical problems that compound severe distress among affected veterans—distress that worsens over time—and the lack of consensus among the experts and authorities over appropriate benefits and compensation (Rand 2008; Finley 2011).

In an attempt to improve services provided to PTSD sufferers, in the 1990s, the Israeli RDMD established a steering committee to assess methods of evaluating psychological disability (Bleich et al. 1993).[18] The committee found that the evaluation criteria in place did not reflect the full range of functional and readjustment difficulties stemming from cognitive, emotional, social, and somatic impairments caused by PTSD.[19] The steering committee recommended instituting a multidisciplinary evaluation model that would reflect the entire range of functional impairment experienced by veterans. These steering committee recommendations were submitted two and a half years before Solomon and Bleich found that the disability ratings assigned by the RDMD are too low and fail to reflect the severity of the veterans' psychological conditions and functional impairments (Bleich & Solomon 2002). In other words, although the Ministry of Defense officially adopted the committee's recommendations, the testimonies and data presented by experts to the Goren Committee in 2010 show that they were not fully implemented, if at all.

Of course, difficulties always arise when trying to change the attitudes of service providers in an institution as large as Ministry of Defense. However, a comprehensive review of the relevant material by the author demonstrates that the more significant reasons for nonimplementation of the Committee's recommendations were related to efforts at economizing and to the persistence of prejudice. From a medical point of view, those suffering from war trauma are considered by the defense establishment as lightly wounded, needing no lifesaving procedures, yet they are costly consumers of the system's financial and human resources, and the expenditure required for their often lengthy treatment is a burden on the system (Rubenstein 2008).[20] The negative labeling of the psychologically traumatized—a phenomenon that has yet to disappear in Israel and elsewhere—and the suspicion of "compensation neurosis"—that is, exaggerating or faking symptoms, of which the PTSD victims are often suspected—support the defense establishment's desire to economize by weeding out potential patients who would cost the government money for years. The two phenomena are intertwined, producing a circle of labeling and economizing.

Many of those who regard trauma claimants with suspicion claim that the psychologically traumatized are, by and large, more interested in benefits than in psychological treatment and that compensation itself poses an obstacle to their recovery, inasmuch as recovery would render the compensation superfluous. Prejudices against claimants were crudely demonstrated in early writing on post-trauma, suggesting that psychological reactions to trauma appear only in cases where there is a prospect of compensation, due to a "conscious or unconscious attempt to elicit monetary benefits" (Solomon et al. 1994). Solomon and her colleagues cite scholarly opinions of the 1980s, which equate disability benefits to a "prospect of an economic windfall," and claimed that this unexpected income encouraged magical thinking, discouraged individual autonomy, and was a motivation to avoid work. According to these views, when the patient realizes, after receiving compensation, that the settlement is inadequate and is even accompanied by a degree of social stigma with it, his condition worsens.[21] This attitude reflects a common hostility toward trauma sufferers and a view of compensation as a "bonanza," tantamount to winning the lottery, rather than reimbursement for the claimant's suffering, loss of his previous life, and his diminished ability to earn a living. This prejudicial attitude is evident in Israel as elsewhere, albeit tempered by therapeutic claims. From within the IDF and Defense Ministry rehabilitation system one currently hears the argument that financial assistance undermines the motivation to recover and regain the ability to function in the workplace to some degree.[22] The desire for compensation, so the argument goes, "taints" the treatment. Those who hold this view see as evidence the fact that only a minority of those referred for treatment see it through, as well as of the fact that some veterans do not claim benefits—something they interpret as based on the fact that "what they really want is treatment."[23]

This attitude—that compensation works as an incentive to avoid recovery—does contain a grain of truth. A number of researchers have posited that the link between the benefits system and the treatment system may indeed disrupt the recovery process, and that the fact that psychotherapy constitutes part of the process by which soldiers apply to receive benefits has implications for the therapy itself. When a patient already troubled by numerous functional impairments is faced with the possibility of a cutback in benefits, it can dissuade him from exhibiting behavior or pursuing a course of action that might be interpreted as an improvement in his or her condition. But when considering the merits of this argument, one must also consider the cyclical nature of PTSD, in which periods of improvement and periods of regression often repeatedly succeed each other. It is only natural that trauma sufferers would fear that any improvement in their condition is temporary and that they might lose their benefits despite being incapable of holding down a job in the long term. Indeed, based on recommendations of professional health care providers, the aforementioned Hasson Committee has proposed a bill that would make permanent the disability ratings assigned to veterans recognized as suffering from PTSD. Advocates of this proposal maintain that it would free these patients from the fear of financial hardship and enable them to focus on their therapy and their recovery efforts.[24]

Equally problematic is the argument that treatment noncompliance or nonadherence reflects a lack of desire to recover. This argument ignores other subjective and objective difficulties that cause many trauma sufferers to periodically drop out of treatment, whether because they feel it is not helping them or because they believe they should learn to "live with their problems."[25] This phenomenon is well known in other armies in the world. In the US army, for example, a report of a Mental Health Advisory Team of 2003 revealed that many soldiers find it hard to get time off from work to seek care, and that 59% of service members fear that mental health care would result in their being seen as weak (Finley 2011). Moreover, in Israel therapy noncompliance is increasingly observed among those traumatized veterans who do not file claims with the RDMD altogether, rather than among veterans who receive benefits (Solomon & Bleich 2002). This claim that disability benefits serve as an incentive to avoid treatment is inconsistent also with the fact that the RDMD limits the number of therapy sessions available to trauma sufferers. There is an inner contradiction between the blame of not seeing through a (long-term) therapy process and the RDMD limit on financing such therapy processes, as well as its position that "recovery-oriented therapy with recovery goals and objectives need not be provided for long periods of time."[26]

However doubtful the anti-benefits arguments may be, the grain of truth on which they are based and the need for traumatized veterans to cope with it call for a practical response from experts in the field. As shown earlier, mental health care professionals have made several suggestions to deal with this problem: effecting a complete separation between the medical committees and treatment services and the system of benefits distribution so as to ensure treatment, and regardless of a veteran's classification for compensation purposes, develop a rehabilitation model that not only is medico-therapeutic but also includes a social dimension.[27]

However, these proposals have yet to be approved, and the dominant discourse in the Defense Ministry remains one of suspicion, with the psychologically traumatized often viewed as "potential exaggerators" (Bleich & Solomon 2002, p. 50). This attitude stands in complete contrast to both Israeli and American data, which clearly obviate the need for suspicion and indicate a low rate of exaggeration and dissimulation. The Israeli data actually prove that those IDF veterans afflicted with CSR and PTSD who seek compensation generally do so only in the absence of any alternative (Solomon & Bleich 2002). A study that compared a group of benefit recipients with a control group of traumatized veterans receiving no financial compensation found that the sole factor that consistently distinguished the two groups was the degree of symptom severity and functional disability. Benefit recipients experienced greater traumatic stress than those in the control group, resulting in higher levels of impairment. The study showed no difference between the benefits group and the control group in terms of their prewar personal attributes. The two groups received similar ratings on all military assessments of their physical and intellectual skills, and psychological fitness for military service. In fact, prewar assessments of adjustment potential of the benefits group were slightly higher than for the control group.[28] In other words, benefit recipients did not suffer from any health or adjustment issues prior to their military service, and there is nothing to indicate that they sought financial compensation as an easy solution to preexisting problems. These findings support the assessment that, in the majority of cases, compensation claims are based on the real needs of claimants whose exposure to trauma was especially intense and whose resulting injury was especially severe, compromising their ability to rebuild their lives. Thus, concludes Professor Zahava Solomon, whose groundbreaking research on CSR and PTSD earned her the Israel Prize for 2009, there is no basis for attributing nonrecovery to a fear of losing benefits: "The financial arrangement afforded no amelioration of their psychological problems; these psychological problems persist, they are severe, complex and extensive."[29] In addition, one must remember that the benefits received by trauma sufferers will never equal the earnings that a healthy person is capable of. None of those who argue that trauma sufferers are excessively dependent on their benefits have explained why young people who had once been energetic, capable, and untroubled by adjustment issues would voluntarily forego all that they might have achieved in life in favor of a limited allowance and a dependent existence.

"Compensation neurosis" bias also appears to be the main factor behind the conduct of the medical committees, which has been criticized not only by the trauma casualties themselves but also by experts in the field. Criticisms against these committees suggest that they overly identify with the defense establishment and are overly concerned with the RDMD's budgetary constraints rather than with purely medical assessments, frequently causing grievous injustice to claimants. These committees have also been accused of disrespectful treatment and degrading attitudes toward trauma sufferers, in violation of the Supreme Court's urging not to "undermine the legislation, which was enacted to benefit the disabled person, and not to subject him to stringencies" (Litman 2007).[30] Solomon's testimony before the Goren Committee paints a troubling picture of the medical committees responsible for assessing CSR and PTSD. According to Solomon, only 3% of returning POWs, the vast majority of whom (90%) are recognized as suffering from PTSD, express satisfaction with the medical committees, while most feel that the committees subjected them to a harsh and humiliating investigative process. Solomon quotes Dr. David Szenes, a clinical psychologist, returning POW, and nephew of Hannah Szenes (an Israeli war hero and female paratrooper trained to rescue Jews during the Holocaust, who was captured and killed by the Nazis): "I underwent three harsh and humiliating investigations. The first during my period of captivity in Egypt, the second on my return to the Zikhron Ya'akov [debriefing] facility, and the third before the Defense Ministry committee."[31] Those afflicted with battle shock—Solomon continues—encounter "both disrespect and a lack of professionalism" because of the very limited knowledge of PTSD among the majority of medical committee members.[32] According to the Association for the Advancement of Combat Stress Reaction Sufferers, the RDMD is so suspicious of PTSD claims that it conducts surveillance of veterans who have already been classified as disabled. Why, then, should one be surprised that these veterans feel persecuted by and distrustful of the RDMD?[33]

The foregoing testimonies and research findings paint a picture of a complicated administrative process, riddled with obstacles, designed to severely restrict eligibility for benefits, and requiring great energy and determination from claimants wishing to pursue it to completion. Because these attributes are not characteristic of trauma sufferers, it would not be groundless to assume that many claimants forego the process altogether. Highly relevant in this regard is a study by Solomon and Mikulincer, who tracked fluctuations in the psychological condition of all soldiers identified as having suffered CSR during the First Lebanon War over a 20-year period. The study also tracked the condition of a control group, veterans of the war with a similar health profile, who were exposed to the same risk situations of CSR but had not been classified as such. The study found that 39% of the control group—who had never sought recognition or compensation from the Defense Ministry for any psychological disability—had suffered from PTSD at various times since the war.[34] What the data imply is that Israel is home to a very large number of people afflicted with war-related PTSD who receive no treatment or assistance from the state.

The Emotional Barrenness of the Insurance-Oriented Discourse

A soldier who is wounded in war experiences a sudden and stark change in the nature of his interaction with the defense establishment. In the blink of an eye, the ideologically charged discourse of heroism and self-sacrifice is replaced by a legalistic discourse of claims and rights. This change takes place at a moment of crisis and disruption of normal life for the soldier. The soldier who prior to the war had likely seen himself and been regarded by others as the very image of independence, strength, and altruism now finds himself wounded and dependent on others. To cope with so radical a change in one's self-image requires support, empathy, and, above all, a renewed sense of meaning and self-worth, as many servicemen afflicted with PTSD have written and stated.[35]

However, instead of pursuing its interactions with wounded soldiers within the context of the same ideologically oriented discourse as before the injury, the RDMD assumes the role of a quasi-insurance company, assessing claims filed against it by soldiers, rather than aiding those injured in the course of their service.[36] Apart from exceptional instances, such as returning POWs, who are automatically eligible for treatment since 1998, the RDMD never contacts wounded veterans at its own initiative but rather leaves them to file their own claims. The very term "claim" signifies an inherent conflict of interests embedded in the relationship between injured veterans and the state, rather than a reciprocal relationship in which the state simply holds up its end of the "bargain," following through on an obligation to its soldiers.[37] This is an agonizing and often humiliating process, in which the wounded veteran bears the burden of demonstrating the scope of his or her impairment and the needs dictated by that impairment. The dissonance between burden of proof imposed on the soldier by these bureaucratic processes post-injury and the heroic discourse that preceded the injury often fills the soldier with disappointment, confusion, and pain. "All the people here [IDF disabled veterans], their lives have changed forever, [and they did it] *for you*," said Major Dubi Ganish, who lost his leg in Lebanon. "All we want is to be free of the burden of proof. [We want] to come here, and have them say, you were wounded in the war, what do you need?" (quoted in Dayan et al. 2009).[38] The severity of the disappointment experienced by these wounded veterans stems from a violation of the principle of reciprocity, which they had understood as the foundation of their relationship with the state. The soldiers sacrificed their health and their previous lives without calculating how much it would "cost" them, and they expect the society to be there for them and to help them regain their lives.

While physically and psychologically wounded soldiers find themselves in similarly inimical relations with the state, further afflictions await the psychologically traumatized. In part because of the invisibility of his wound and the difficulty of proving its existence, the burden of the traumatized soldier also arises from the disorder's very nature. PTSD by definition makes interpersonal communication hard, and these difficulties worsen in conflict situations. These difficulties, along with the need to revisit, as part of the claims process, the very experiences and memories that the trauma sufferer ordinarily prefers not to reawaken, pose the risk of temporarily intensifying the patient's PTSD symptoms (Bleich & Solomon 2002).

Many physically wounded veterans also suffer from psychological trauma, but typically receive treatment only for their physical injuries. Data presented by

Chaim Knobler to the Goren Committee show that although the prevalence of CSR among physically wounded veterans is much higher than among the non-wounded, only a small proportion of the physically wounded have been classified by the RDMD as having suffered psychological trauma.[39] In other words, even in the case of soldiers whose visible wounds are recognized by the state, the bloodless wound is left to fester, unacknowledged.

Studies have shown that the chance of suffering from CSR directly correlates with a soldier's sense of isolation, which may emerge on the battlefield in inverse proportion to the support provided by commanding officers. The impact of isolation is so great that it offers the best single predictor of CSR (Solomon et al. 1987). By extension, one can link this risk factor to the feelings experienced by soldiers during their postinjury interactions with military and medical bureaucracy. These feelings frequently include alienation and a lack of support from the military and society as a whole. This intensified sense of isolation compromises the ability of veterans afflicted with PTSD to cope with their condition.

Lack of support, however, is not an unfounded feeling on the part of veterans. When senior military officials still cast doubt on the very legitimacy of the psychological trauma diagnosis, soldiers feel abandoned. A striking example is the statement by Brigadier General Avigdor Kahalani, who, during the Goren Committee deliberations, declared, "every soldier who has fought on the battlefield has PTSD . . . So it's hard to make the distinction, and we see there are people who are able to get mileage out of it since they don't have to show a bleeding arm."[40] Kahalani's statement reflects the common, though ignorant, belief that there is no difference between CSR and the ordinary challenges of the battlefield experienced by all soldiers. It also points to the stubborn persistence of the notion that recognizing trauma depletes morale and that an ethos of heroism can render soldiers immune. The idea that soldiers can be expected to "normalize" their psychological trauma and write it off as just another difficult war experience is reminiscent of the attitudes toward CSR sufferers during the early decades of Israel's statehood. It also reveals the degree to which progress in understanding the phenomenon remains offset by rigid and conservative views regarding the role of the individual in society.

Wounded veterans testify to having harbored the expectation that society would welcome them with open arms on their return from the front. In their unrequited yearning, one hears echoes of the frustration and disappointment experienced by another group of people in a very different time and place and under profoundly different conditions: the quarter of a million Holocaust survivors interned in displaced persons camps in Germany, Austria, and Italy after World War II. The dissimilarities notwithstanding, in each case a group of people traumatized in the context of national conflict sought relief from national representatives. Despite significant success with practical assistance, the survivors' encounter with the emissaries from Eretz Yisrael[41] was rife with disappointment, loneliness, and a sense that their emotional needs had not been met (Keynan 1996). As one observer put it in the newspaper *HaNitzotz* in 1947, "The power of the delegation should have consisted . . . in an inherently paternal attitude. The inner distress, in which many of the 'surviving remnants' were mired, needed to be eased . . . Emotional life [had to be] restored to its normal path, if only partially. The 'surviving remnant' was expecting people who would provide solace, embrace them, guide them and be . . . bone of their bone and flesh of their flesh" (Scheinzon 1947, pp. 13–14). Obviously, there are drastic differences between the two historical circumstances, and no attempt to compare them is intended here. Yet even when taking the differences into account, one can identify in both situations the same expectation and longing for a welcoming national embrace among the traumatized.

Citizens of democratic countries ascribe quasi-parental roles to the state, and they therefore expect more than mere financial or technical assistance when injured in service of the state. They expect displays of empathy. Expectations such as these have not declined, despite diminishing levels of trust in governments around the world. Scholars have shown that the reverse is actually true and that current distrust of government stems, in large part, from a tendency to idealize the democratic system (Miller & Listhaug 1999). Moreover, a tendency to attach greater importance to individual rather than collectivist needs and desires—a trend that has been intensifying in Israel since the 1980s—has heightened expectations of reciprocity between the state and its citizens (Yogev 1999).

With such elevated expectations, can the aforementioned individual needs ever be satisfied? The state provides a natural target for anger, an emotion that is easier to bear than mourning and profound sorrow and whose expression provides some relief. For this reason, the state is "always at fault" in the eyes of the wounded (Dayan et al. 2009).[42] However, in contrast to the prevailing view that it is neither possible nor desirable to satisfy what are considered the unrealistic desires of wounded veterans, therapists maintain that the very attempt by state agencies to meet these veterans' needs mitigates their anger and bitterness, and strengthens their ability to cope with their condition.[43]

Furthermore, soldiers raise concrete demands and do not limit their criticism to general feelings of disappointment and sadness. For example, they expect the Ministry of Defense to assume the responsibility for their rehabilitation process. "If I didn't have to be the one to declare that I'm in distress, if it were only obvious, and if they showed some understanding toward a severely traumatized person . . . it would be easier for me," writes Amos Levitov, a POW who spent three and a half years in captivity in Egypt, at the conclusion of his memoir, *The Lie of Silence* (Levitov 2007, p. 159). "No one will come to you," says the wife of a Second Lebanon War veteran afflicted with PTSD. "You have to take the initiative . . . you have to demand" (Efrat, quoted by Dayan et al. 2009). This describes the general pattern of interactions in which the RDMD views itself as an insurance agency, and thereby makes the wounded veterans feel as beggars at the gate.

What emerges is a painful situation in which the psychologically wounded confront a system that is insufficiently sensitive to their plight, and find themselves in a cold, cruel field of adversarial negotiations over their own needs and rights. On these rocks of discourse of contracts and laws, the previously ideological and moral discourse on behalf of which the soldiers were sent to war is now smashed. The complicated deliberations over rights and needs never end. The array of services that the RDMD makes available to wounded veterans, incomplete to begin with, becomes increasingly inadequate to satisfy the veterans' growing needs over time as their functional problems increase in complexity.[44] As Professor Yossi Zohar, director of Sheba Medical Center's Psychiatric Division and chair of the Israeli Consortium on PTSD, illustrated to the Goren Committee, the functional level of PTSD sufferers declines over the years, even with treatment.[45] Some experts blame the treatment modality or the patients' dependence on benefits. But few would challenge the fact that PTSD is a serious illness that responds poorly to treatment, whose symptoms worsen over the years, frequently accompanied by additional physical and mental disorders.[46] It is true that veterans can request a reevaluation by the medical committee, but the committees do not typically increase compensation packages, and the experience of returning to them is harsh and often humiliating.[47]

The levels of distress reported by wounded veterans might seem disproportionate to the bureaucratic frustrations and insufficiencies in services they encounter. A deeper source of their pain, however, is the transformation of their relationship with their country into a series of financial and technical negotiations, in which the veteran is always the weaker party. To a certain degree, the legal and insurance-oriented discourse empties the legitimization of CSR and PTSD of any therapeutic potential. While financial compensation and assistance are necessary, they address only one area of need. For both the trauma sufferers and their families, recognition is the "key concept, one more important than money," and a crucial precondition for soldiers seeking to overcome their emotional wounds (Peled 1999). The post-traumatic experience sets off an identity crisis firmly rooted in a sociocultural context. The greater the soldiers' identification with the IDF and the state, the greater their need for formal recognition of a kind that gives meaning to their suffering and enables them to preserve the portion of themselves that rests on that identification. Therapists maintain that this is one of the reasons why traumatized veterans drop out of treatment once they obtain official recognition that they suffer from PTSD. The recognition itself is a therapeutic force (Cohen & Farsha 2008).

The current format of the traumatized soldier's relationship with the defense establishment does not allow expression of the emotional aspects of recognition, even when it is granted, and therefore these soldiers remain isolated in a state of emotional distress and despair. "I'm in a hole," says Uri Lerner, a PTSD sufferer decorated for having evacuated wounded comrades under fire during the Second Lebanon War. "I want to get out but they won't let me" (quoted in Dayan et al. 2009).

In conclusion, there is an urgent need to stop the insurance-oriented discourse that causes damage to all facets of the relationship between the wounded and the defense establishment. The insurance discourse contains an ingrained, predisposed suspicion of claimants' attempts to claim benefits under false pretenses; it places the soldier in conflict with the very system that is expected to provide warm, loving support; and it juxtaposes potentially healing treatment issues with haggling over the fine print of suffering. It is, moreover, vital to accelerate current efforts to improve treatment methods and facilitate trauma sufferers' interactions with state bureaucracy in ways consistent with the proposals suggested by Zehava Solomon, Chaim Knobler, Itamar Barnea, and others: uncouple the benefits system and the treatment system, and develop models for social, as well as therapeutic, rehabilitation, in conjunction with relevant organizations and self-help groups.

Notes

1. Yoram Kupermintz, a soldier afflicted with battle shock in the Yom Kippur War, quoted by Peled (1999).
2. The unit was founded on the initiative of the Disabled Rehabilitation Division in the Ministry of Defense, and with the cooperation of the chief medical officer (author's interview with Major Dr. Ofir Levy, head of the IDF's CSR Unit, 3 December 2009).
3. The responsibility for discharged soldiers was transferred to the unit from the Ministry of Defense (Shklar 1990; Bleich & Melamed 2007).
4. Disability Item 34A in the List of Diseases, Impairments and Injuries that Confer Recognition of Disability for Wounded IDF Servicemen (Bleich & Melamed 2007).
5. As per author's interview with Miri Shalit, 2009, and conversation with Avi Bleich, chair of NATAL's Steering Committee, 21 May 2009.
6. Levy interview, 2009. Lieutenant-Colonel Dr. Ofir Levy notes that 45% of those currently being treated by the CSR Unit (2009) were injured in earlier wars, including the Six-Day War in 1967.
7. Goren Committee protocol, Chaim Knobler's testimony, 4 March 2010. Available from www.vaadatgoren.gov.il/Portals/0/docs/Goren002.pdf (henceforth "Goren Committee"). Dr. Chaim Knobler served as chief psychiatrist in the IDF; after his discharge in 2005 he founded, with colleagues, the Association for the Advancement of Combat Stress Reaction Sufferers. The way in which responsibility for treatment of CSR sufferers is divided between the CSR Unit and the Defense Ministry changes from time to time.
8. On soldiers' perceptions in this regard, see Dayan et al. (2009).
9. CD/IK confidential interview, 2009.
10. As noted by Saar Uziely in a conversation held by the author with members of the NATAL steering committee, 2 November 2009.
11. See the wounded IDF veterans' demonstration before the Dan and Tel Aviv District Rehabilitation Office at Tel Hashomer, 2 November 2009. The demonstrators were protesting what they referred to as "rehabilitation trauma," an offensive attitude and a failure on the Defense Ministry's part to respect agreements. From www.ynet.co.il/articles/0,7340,L-3799344,00.html, retrieved on 25 July 2010.
12. Information obtained from author's interviews with Major Dr. Ofir Levy (3 December 2009) and Miri Shalit (June 2011), as well as Ministry of Defense (2013).
13. The team appointed by the Knesset to investigate the functional status of the Defense Ministry's Disabled Rehabilitation Division was established during the 18th Knesset by the Foreign Affairs and Defense Committee. The team's interim conclusions (published in February 2010; "The Hasson Committee, Interim Report") and related deliberations can be viewed on Knesset Member Yisrael Hasson's website. Also available on the website are bills aimed at introducing change into the Defense Ministry's Disabled Rehabilitation Division. Retrieved on 12 June 2011 from www.israel-hason.com/subjects_tmp1.asp. The foregoing is based on the author's conversation with MK Yisrael Hasson on 13 February 2011.

14. Tanielian and Jaycox (2008) found a 14% depression rate among soldiers returning from Iraq and Afghanistan, in addition to the 14% who returned with PTSD.
15. Letter of nomination, signed by the prime minister and the minister of defense, 18 November 2009. Available from http://www.vaadatgoren.gov.il/tabid/59/Default.aspx.
16. The Goren Committee, Colonel (Dr.) Knobler's testimony, p. 10. Emphasis mine.
17. See particularly statements by Lt. Col. Stephane Grenier and by the narrator in the film's opening sequence: "If you die they'll salute you and honor your memory every year. If you come back psychologically wounded, they'll discard you like an old rag."
18. The committee was headed by Professor Avi Bleich; committee members included senior psychiatrists as well as Rehabilitation Division personnel in charge of medical, rehabilitation, and medical screening issues.
19. For details on the range of difficulties, see Bleich and Solomon (2002).
20. The term "resource consumer" is per Rubenstein's usage. Although Rubenstein's study deals with the years leading up to the First Lebanon War, his assessment of the situation is still applicable.
21. Solomon et al. (1994) cite D. J. Sprehe, 1984, 'Workers' Compensation: a Psychiatric Follow-Up Study', *International Journal of Law and Psychiatry*, vol. 7, pp. 165–178.
22. Shalit interview, 2009.
23. Levy interview, 2009.
24. Author's conversation with NATAL's chief psychologist, Dr. Itamar Barnea, 16 April 2011. Barnea, a fighter pilot in the Yom Kippur war who was taken prisoner by the Syrians, went on to serve as the chief psychologist of the Israel Air Force and as head of the IDF's Casualties Department (henceforth "Barnea interview, April 2011"). Also: author's correspondence with Miri Shalit, director of Rehabilitation Services in the Disabled Rehabilitation Division's Dan District, June 2011 (henceforth "Shalit correspondence, June 2011"). The issue also came up before the Hasson Committee, which submitted recommendations along these lines to the Ministry of Defense. These recommendations waited for approval when the committee's operations were suspended.
25. Confidential testimony IK/KS, 2009.
26. The Goren Committee, testimony of Zeev Weissman, deputy director of the Disabled Rehabilitation Division in the Ministry of Defense, within the framework of Dr. Knobler's appearance before the Committee.
27. On separating benefits from treatment: Barnea interview, April 2011. Barnea proposes that, within the process of recognition for treatment purposes—to be completely detached from the process of recognition-for-compensation-purposes—the sole area of assessment be the connection between claimant distress and the precipitating security incident, and that this assessment be carried out by a professional party (a psychologist or social worker), rather than by a medical committee, and without reference to the degree of impairment. Should a connection be found, the claimant should be entitled to a three-year course of treatment, independent of the recognition-for-compensation-purposes process. On shortening the application process: Miri Shalit, director of Rehabilitation Services in the Disabled Rehabilitation Division's Dan District, and Itamar Barnea, NATAL's chief psychologist, feel that a three-month period is sufficient to establish the presence of chronic PTSD. In their view, lengthening the application process hurts claimants' chances of recovery (Shalit correspondence, June 2011; Barnea interview, April 2011). On shifting the responsibility for veteran therapy to the CSR unit: Goren Committee, Statement of Col. Chaim Knobler, Goren Committee deliberations; Yisrael Hasson interview, 2011. On the social rehabilitation model: Goren Committee, Statement of Zahava Solomon.
28. This refers to the fact that fewer members of the benefits-recipient group reported psychological problems, and fewer of them had any kind of psychiatric diagnosis at the time of their conscription (Solomon & Bleich 2002, p. 177).

29. Goren Committee, Statement of Zahava Solomon, p. 11.
30. Regarding criticism of how the medical committees function, see also Hasson Committee, Interim Report.
31. Goren Committee, Statement of Zahava Solomon, p. 9.
32. Ibid., p. 10.
33. Goren Committee, Statement of Col. (Dr.) Chaim Knobler, p. 11.
34. Goren Committee, Statement of Zehava Solomon. Four percent of these veterans were diagnosed with the syndrome in all four assessments conducted over the years, 6% in three of the assessments, 12% twice, and 17% once; statistics based on Solomon and Mikulincer (2006).
35. See I. Bachar, 2005, *This Is What I Remember*, Kinneret Zmora-Bitan Dvir, Or Yehuda; Ansbacher (2007).
36. Shalit interview, 2009.
37. The problematic nature of the term "claim" and of the rest of the terminology used by the Disabled Rehabilitation Division also came up during the Hasson Committee deliberations; in its interim report the Committee recommended that the matter be subjected to a thoroughgoing investigation. See Hasson Committee, Interim Report.
38. The feeling that wounded veterans are perceived as a burden on society and on the state has also been expressed by treatment providers. See statement by Judith Yovel Recanati, Chair of NATAL, in the author's conversation with NATAL Steering Committee members, 2 November 2009.
39. Goren Committee, Statement of Col. (Dr.) Knobler, p. 12. Knobler cites a study by Professor Ehud Klein.
40. Goren Committee, Statement of Brigadier General Avigdor Kahalani, member of the Committee, during Zahava Solomon's appearance before the Committee, p. 18. See also transcript of Kuti Mor's testimony before the Goren Committee during the discussion of disease and PTSD caused by events during reserve duty: "Let me tell you, the 'personal effort' method usually works. If I succeed, great. If I don't succeed, I try again."
41. Eretz Yisrael, the land of Israel, is the Hebrew name Jews used for the area of the British Mandate (1922–1948), until the birth of the State of Israel. The name comes from the Bible, the territory that God promised to Abraham. In other languages is also called the Promised Land, or the Holy Land and the Land of Milk and Honey.
42. Quotes were taken from a question directed toward interviewees by Ilana Dayan: "Could it be that the state has no chance with you?" and "Could it be that it's always to blame?"
43. Author's conversation with members of the NATAL Steering Committee, 2 November 2009. Statement of Sigal Haimov.
44. One example: the size of the monthly allowance paid to veterans whose disability rating is 100% (i.e., who are unable to work) does not take into consideration the difference between the earning ability and necessities of life of a 20-year-old soldier and those of a man at the height of his career. Confidential testimony IK/BI, 2009.
45. Goren Committee, Professor Zohar's testimony. See also slides 11–12 of Zohar's presentation to the Committee.
46. Goren Committee, Statement of Zahava Solomon, p. 4, and Slide 6 of her presentation.
47. Confidential communication with a veteran who was recognized as suffering from PTSD 40 years ago. IK/SD, 2013.

References

American Psychological Association 2013, *DSM-5 Posttraumatic Stress Disorder Fact Sheet.* Available from www.dsm5.org/Documents/PTSD%20Fact%20Sheet.pdf.

Ansbacher, M. 2007, *Fragment of the Silver Platter*, Daniella De-Nur, Tel Aviv (Hebrew)

Bleich, A., Bar-Natan, A., Schlossberg, A., Laor, G., Dolfin, D., Galzhavsky, V., & Arel, Y. 1993, 'Concluding Report', Psychiatric Steering Committee, Disabled Rehabilitation Division, Ministry of Defense. Available from http://ptsdil.info [19 August 2011].

Bleich, A., & Melamed, Y. 2007, 'Post-Traumatic Emotional Damage and Impairment Following Military Service', *Journal of Medicine and Law*, vol. 37, pp. 37–44. (Hebrew)

Bleich, A., & Solomon, Z. 2002, 'Evaluating Psychological Disability—Conceptual and Clinical Issues' in *Mental Disability: Medical, Research Social, Legal and Rehabilitative Aspects*, eds. A. Bleich & Z. Solomon, Ministry of Defense, Tel Aviv, pp. 26–39. (Hebrew)

Cohen, M., & Farsha, E. 2008, 'Social and Cultural Contexts of Combat Stress Reaction: War Trauma as Identity Crisis', *Hebrew Psychology* [electronic version]. Available from www.hebpsy.net/articles.asp?id-1781 [27 July 2010]. (Hebrew)

Dayan, I., Tokatli, G., & Asenheim, O. 2009, 'Forsaken Heroes', *Uvda*, Keshet Broadcasting, 23 March.

The Disabled Law (Benefits and Rehabilitation), Amendment No. 21 (Psychological Disability and Battle Shock), 2000, Israel.

Finley, E. 2011, *Fields of Combat, Understanding PTSD among Veterans of Iraq and Afghanistan*, Cornell University Press, Ithaca.

Inbar, D., Solomon, Z., Aviram, U., & Spiro, S. 1989, 'Officers' Attitudes toward Combat Stress Reaction: Responsibility, Treatment, Return to Unit, and Personal Distance', *Mil. Med.*, vol. 159, no. 9, pp. 480–487.

Keynan, I. 1996, *The Hunger Has Not Abated: the Surviving Remnants of the Holocaust and the Israeli Pre-State Emissaries, 1945–1948*, Am Oved Press, Tel Aviv. (Hebrew)

Levitov, A. 2007, *The Lie of Silence*, Ministry of Defense, Tel Aviv.

Litman, S. 2007, Editor's note on the article by A. Bleich & Y. Melamed, 'Post-Traumatic Psychological Impairment Subsequent to Military Service', *Refuah vMishpat* [Law and medicine], vol. 37, p. 44. (Hebrew)

Miller, A., & Listhaug, O. 1999, 'Political Performance and Institutional Trust' in *Critical Citizens, Global Support for Democratic Governance*, ed. P. Norris, Oxford University Press, Oxford, pp. 204–216.

Ministry of Defense (Israel), 2013, 'Rights of Disabled IDF Veterans', June. Available from www.shikum.mod.gov.il/shikumh/UploadDocs/ZakayInfo.pdf [12 April 2014].

Moering, R. G. 2011, 'Military Service Records: Searching for the Truth', *Psychological Injury and Law*, vol. 4, pp. 217–234.

Operation Retour 2005, documentary film.

Peled, A. 1999, 'No Signs of Shock Were Found', *Yedioth Ahronoth*, *7 Days* supplement, 6 August.

Rand Center for Military Health Policy Research 2008, 'Invisible Wounds of War'. Available from www.rand.org/content/dam/rand/pubs/monographs/2008/RAND_MG720.pdf.

Rubenstein, Z. 2008, *From Battle Shock to Combat Stress Reaction: a History of Paradigm Change in the Yom Kippur and Lebanon Wars, as Reflected in the Care-Provider and Mental Health Systems Narrative*, doctoral dissertation, Tel Aviv University. (Hebrew)

Scheinzon, Y. D. 1947, 'The Urgent Problems of the Surviving Remnant', *HaNitzotz*, vol. 73, no. 6, pp. 13–14.

Shalom, D., Benbenishty, R., & Solomon, Z. 1995, 'Mental Health Officers' Causal Explanations of Combat Stress Reaction', *Journal of Traumatic Stress*, vol. 8, no. 2, pp. 259–269.

Shklar, R. 1990, 'Mental Health in Uniform—the Development of the IDF's Mental Health System', *Bit'on Hel HaRefuah* [I.D.F. Medical Corps bulletin], vol. 32, pp. 5–7.

Skodol, A. E., Schwartz, S., Dohrenwend, B. P., Levav, I., Shrout, P. E., & Reiff, M. 1996, 'PTSD Symptoms and Comorbid Mental Disorders in Israeli War Veterans', *British Journal of Psychiatry*, vol. 169, pp. 717–725.

Solomon, Z. 1993, *Combat Stress Reaction, the Enduring Toll of War*, Plenum Press, New York.

Solomon, Z., Benbenishty, R., Waysman, M., & Bleich, A. 1994, 'Compensation and Psychic Trauma: a Study of Israeli Combat Veterans', *American Journal of Orthopsychiatry*, vol. 64, no. 1, pp. 91–102.

Solomon, Z. & Bleich, A. 2002, 'Psychological Disability and the Compensation Claim—Potential Reciprocal Influences' in *Mental Disability: Medical, Research Social, Legal and Rehabilitative Aspects*, eds. A. Bleich & Z. Solomon, Ministry of Defense, Tel Aviv, pp. 163–197. (Hebrew)

Solomon, Z., & Mikulincer, M. 2006, 'Trajectories of PTSD: a 20-Year Longitudinal Study', *American Journal of Psychiatry*, vol. 163, pp. 659–666.

Solomon, Z., Mikulincer, M., & Hobfoll, S. 1987, 'Battle Intensity, Social Support, Loneliness and Combat Reactions: the Israeli Experience in the Lebanon War', *Society and Welfare*, vol. 5, no. 2, pp. 114–127. (Hebrew)

Tanielian, T., & Jaycox, L. H. 2008, *Invisible Wounds of War: Psychological and Cognitive Injuries, Their Consequences and Services to Assist Recovery*, Rand, Santa Monica, CA.

Worthen, M., & Moering, R. 2011, 'A Practical Guide to Conducting VA Compensation and Pension Exams for PTSD and Other Mental Disorders', *Psychological Injury and Law*, vol. 4, no. 3–4, pp. 187–216.

Yogev, A. 1999, 'Order in the Chaos: Israeli Education Policy in the Post-Modern Era' in *Public Policy in Israel*, eds. D. Nachmias & G. Menachem, Israel Democracy Institute, Jerusalem. (Hebrew)

5 Trauma and War Debate in Israel

Doubts over a Needless Sacrifice

The First Lebanon War (1982) was controversial from the outset. A "war of choice," it seemed to run counter to the prevailing Israeli ethos, according to which the country went to war only when there was no other choice.[1] Prime Minister Menachem Begin had announced that the campaign's objective was to advance no more than 40 kilometers (25 miles) into Lebanon. Therefore, when Defense Minister Ariel Sharon's plan to conquer Beirut became known, many Israelis felt they had been deceived by the government, calling into question, for the first time in the country's history, the necessity of hundreds of Israeli casualties. An expression began to permeate Israeli public discourse that had never been heard before: "a needless war," a war unworthy of its sacrifices.

The term "needless," harsh and unfamiliar to Israeli ears in matters of national security, had first gained currency nine years earlier, during the Yom Kippur War. However, those who employed it at the time applied it to the scope of Israeli losses, which, they believed, could have been diminished had Israel not blundered into war unprepared.[2] During the First Lebanon War the term took on a new, more troubling meaning that reflected the absence of the small solace of national existential necessity. Bereaved families who opposed the war were tormented by the purposelessness of their loss, whereas those who had believed in the war's necessity were tormented by a loss voided of meaning.[3] Whatever their similarities in terms of pain, the stark differences among the families of the fallen could not be masked. "One father laments the falling of his son in a war that he regards as unjustified, and suffers bitterly," declared the famous author Yizhar Smilansky at the unveiling of a memorial at Tel Aviv University. "Another father laments the falling of his son in that same war and does not accept that the war is being called unnecessary: his son died in the nation's war for peace in the Galilee, and he suffers bitterly."[4]

The First Lebanon War also forced Israeli society to openly confront doubts previously repressed regarding Israel Defense Forces (IDF)'s "purity of arms," the belief that the army always exercised restraint in its use of force and that it resorted to violence only when necessary, avoiding hurting civilians, even at the risk of losing soldiers. The public was divided between those who awoke in June 1982 to an undermined national ethos and wondered where they could "hide the shame" (Oz 1982) and those who justified, and still justify today, the bombing of a civilian population on the grounds that it was necessary "for our survival" (Megged 1982). The doubts expressed in Israeli national discourse about the IDF's purity of arms escalated in the wake of the Sabra and Shatila massacre, which shook the Israeli public to its core. Profound controversy ensued over the degree of responsibility borne by Israel for the slaughter of hundreds of Palestinian inhabitants of refugee camps by Lebanese Christian Phalangist forces within territory controlled by the IDF. In 1982, after 15 years of Israeli rule in the Occupied Territories (henceforth the territories),[5] the country had a growing familiarity with the Palestinian population. This repeated encounter with a civilian population in distress—this time in Lebanon—made it impossible to retain the image of a faceless and nameless enemy, necessary to avoid empathizing with their suffering and to preserve the myth of purity of arms (Kashti & Rimon Or 1999). The recent peace treaty with Egypt (1979) may also have cast doubt on the belief that the conflict could never be resolved by peaceful means.

A fraught public climate thus developed in which opposition to endangering soldiers in unnecessary wars merged with a growing debate over proportionality of force and harming civilian populations. Doubt regarding the war's necessity became exacerbated by concern over the justness of the cause. The escalating wave of dissent took on new and unfamiliar forms as soldiers and bereaved parents threw off the shackles of convention and cooperated in the shattering of myths. Reserve soldiers sang macabre protest songs about dying in war at the whim of their leaders, dozens refused the call-up for reserve duty, and bereaved parents unhesitatingly protested the harm suffered by Lebanese civilians.[6] In "Children," a poem that appeared in the 1983 anthology *Border Crossing*, commissioned, in part, by bereaved parents, Ephraim Sidon warned, "As you've been briefed/When bringing chocolate to a wounded child/Make sure he still has lips/So he can thank you with a smile" (Sidon 1983).[7]

The deep divisions and sense of needless loss that characterized the Israeli response to the First Lebanon War marked an upsurge in rates of CSR among IDF soldiers. Nearly a quarter of those wounded in the war suffered from CSR, and as delayed reactions set in, their numbers increased threefold over the following decade (Neria et al. 1998). According to data compiled by the Israeli Consortium on PTSD, the number of veterans who suffered PTSD from serving in the First Lebanon War is nearly identical to the number from the much larger-scale Yom Kippur war.[8] At first glance this figure seems surprising, given the circumstances of the Yom Kippur War, which greatly increased the risk of developing CSR. The Yom Kippur War hit the Israeli public with no warning, profoundly undermined IDF soldiers' trust in military and political leadership, and thrust many soldiers into combat situations where they had virtually no chance of survival. The First Lebanon War, on the other hand, was relatively small in scale. Harsh though many of the battles were, in only a few of them did soldiers experience the kind of hopelessness common during the 1973 war.

Yet the prevalence of CSR among soldiers in the First Lebanon War is less surprising when one takes into account the importance of social support and believing in the goals of a given war in preventing CSR. The Lebanon War ushered in a new era of perpetual debate about the goals of war. It also marked the transition from traditional warfare between armies, which had characterized all of Israel's previous wars, to conflict with guerilla organizations operating from within a civilian population. The changing character of fighting conditions provoked a change in attitude toward war itself and toward the IDF. Since the Yom Kippur War, no war or military action undertaken by Israel has enjoyed national consensus. Even in those instances where support for military action has been relatively broad, such as Operation Cast Lead in 2008, the public did not regard these campaigns as "wars of no choice." Thus did Israel abandon a principle that had dominated the country's understanding of war during its first quarter-century of existence: war was a last resort.

The bitter disputes now occasioned by all military actions and by the changing character of warfare in general expose the IDF to constant domestic criticism and make it harder for soldiers to cope with the ambiguous face of the enemy. The responsibility that the Israeli public places on the IDF has, since the 1980s, been complicated by contradictory demands. Public opinion of the military swings back and forth, like a pendulum. Even when a military operation elicits wide public support, such consensus quickly erodes once the IDF has suffered its first losses in battle or when the media outlets report large-scale harm to Palestinian civilians. At that point, public debate heats up, and the army finds itself under attack domestically and internationally. In a way, this is a reflection of the discrepancy familiar from the literature on military ethics between *jus ad bellum* and *jus in bello*. The former refers to the criteria for justifying war; the latter denotes the acceptability of wartime conduct. Support for a war does not always translate into legitimization of how it is fought (Cook 2001).

These discrepancies and contradictions appeared in Israel for the first time during the First Lebanon War and led to an increase in the number of CSR sufferers. Similar features, with accordingly rising risks of CSR, have characterized Israel's military conflicts from that point on.

Moral Injury—The Transparent Trauma[9]

The nature of war is that every soldier is both the potential victim and agent of violence. The denial of the existence of war trauma, however common in cases when soldiers are victims, is even more prevalent when discussing soldiers traumatized by committing violence, particularly when civilians have been harmed. The international literature refers to such soldiers as "self-traumatized perpetrators," meaning that they have been traumatized by participating, directly or indirectly, in acts of violence, especially ones that were ethically problematic. Discussion of this issue raises complex moral questions and elicits strong sentiments. In the US the topic is linked to the controversy over the Vietnam War and to a lack of consensus on the validity or necessity of the PTSD diagnosis per se, a diagnosis that, as noted earlier, was included in the third (1980) edition of the American Psychiatric Association's *Diagnostic and Statistical Manual of Mental Disorders* (DSM-III).[10] Anthropologist Allan Young, a leading critic of the diagnosis, does not deny the existence of PTSD, but rather contends that its DSM definition was formulated to respond to the needs of Vietnam veterans, and that it applies as well to war criminals, those who, having perpetrated atrocities against a civilian population, brought their trauma upon themselves (Young 2002). According to Young, the committee that defined the criteria for diagnosing PTSD addressed the etiological features of traumatic events, rather than the content of these events or the reasons behind the violence. This opened the door to trauma diagnoses for perpetrators of violence, where the trauma resulted from the very fact of having committed an atrocity. This criticism became particularly relevant in the wake of incidents where American soldiers were responsible for the needless slaughter and abuse of Vietnamese civilians. One well-known and extreme incident of this kind was the My Lai massacre, which triggered intensified anti-war protests even outside the US.[11] The indiscriminate slaughter of innocents in My Lai was exceptional in its barbarity, but acts of cruelty and killing of civilians were quite common in the Vietnam War. Once knowledge of these acts penetrated the American public consciousness, the fierce debates—already fueled by the prolonged conflict—began to address the issue of moral responsibility as well. Those who share Allan Young's view see the soldier who commits inappropriate acts as bearing full responsibility. Others place the blame on the war itself or on those responsible for sending the soldiers (Scott 1990). Prominent advocates of this approach include Chaim Shatan and Robert Jay Lifton, distinguished psychiatrists known both for their vehement opposition to the Vietnam War and for spearheading the effort to ensure recognition of the post-traumatic syndrome to which so many veterans of that war succumbed, even helping to formulate its definition in the DSM-III. According to Shatan and Lifton, soldiers who had committed atrocities were themselves victims, forced into this behavior by military and political leaders and, to a certain degree, the American public, which allowed this irrational war to happen. Lifton claimed that conditions in the Vietnam War were "atrocity producing situations" (Lifton 2005; Lifton and Shatan both quoted by Young 2002, pp. 641, 634). Lifton, Shatan, and others regarded the cruelties committed by the soldiers as symbols of the moral bankruptcy of America's involvement in Vietnam. According to them, the psychological conditions that soldiers are subjected to during military training, compounded by the extreme physical and mental exhaustion in wartime, impair their ability to engage in critical thinking. This ability is further limited in ambiguous situations, where the goals of war are unclear and where it is hard to distinguish between enemy and innocent civilian.

At the heart of the debate about the trauma suffered by the inflictor of harm, which cannot be addressed here with appropriate thoroughness, lies the question of moral responsibility. On the one hand, the PTSD diagnosis raises concerns that by recognizing soldiers who have acted with inappropriate violence as injured parties in their own right, we will be transforming these soldiers from criminals into victims, freeing them of personal responsibility for what they have done. On the other hand, doubts about the moral autonomy of soldiers under conditions of stress, fatigue, and danger reaffirm the responsibility borne by military and political policymakers.

When a soldier takes military action against an enemy who has the potential to inflict similar damage, he can function on the battlefield without risk to his beliefs or values. By contrast, atypical military activity in the heart of a civilian population engenders conflict between personal or universal values and moral codes, on the one hand, and the accepted norms of military life, on the other, including the imperative to follow orders and the value placed on loyalty to one's comrades in arms (Hobfoll & Milgram 1986, quoted by Gal 1990). A combat situation in which a soldier participates in the humiliation, abuse, or killing of civilians creates cognitive dissonance between what the soldier regards as legitimate and what he perceives as actually going on, exposing him to pathological stress reactions (ibid.). The weightier the moral dilemma, the more overwhelming the internal conflict and the greater the risk of CSR, even when the soldier perceives the goals of the war as justified. This is especially true when soldiers feel unable to act as their conscience dictates because of a sense of personal danger, uncertainty about the identity or intentions of those whom they are facing, or pressure from commanding officers and fellow servicemen.

A particular difficulty faces IDF soldiers serving in the territories, which are densely populated with civilians. It stems first and foremost from conditions in the field, frequently characterized by a mixture, whether intentional or unintentional, of Palestinian combatants, Hamas and Jihad fighters, and the noncombatant population.

Israeli law provides the soldier with immunity under the rubric of "obedience to orders," according to which he cannot be charged with an offense if he has carried out an illegal order. However, this defense applies only if the order was not "unquestionably illegal," such as committing atrocities, in which case the soldier is expected to disobey.[12] The defense and its conditional nature are meant to address both the soldier's duty to carry out orders and his concomitant duty to refrain from acts on which "should fly, like a black flag, a warning saying: 'Prohibited!'" (Ruling of Judge Benjamin Halevy, Military Prosecutor v. Major Malinki et al. 1957). It would seem that receiving an unquestionably illegal order would be easier for a soldier to handle, since the duty to disobey such an order spares him any moral reflection. Moral reflection is also easier in situations where an order has been received to execute an act that is illegal, but not unquestionably illegal. Relying on the immunity, a soldier can cope with such an order without damaging his sense of moral integrity. What soldiers find harder to contend with are vague and inconsistent orders. Such orders can be interpreted in different ways and force soldiers to weigh their moral and practical consequences under the stressful conditions of a military operation. The moral ambiguity and uncertainty as to whether immunity is applicable in a given instance place the soldier in a state of emotional distress. In such a situation the soldier is liable to carry out orders based on his own interpretation of them, while his commanding officer may later claim that those were not the orders at all.[13] The difficulty posed by vague commands when carrying out operations in a civilian area is nothing new and has accompanied Israeli soldiers since 1948. As Mordechai Gur, the IDF's tenth chief of staff, said while referring to the code of purity of arms formulated by Ben-Gurion and Yitzhak

Sadeh, "The most difficult period of the War of Independence was the one after the battles ended, when refugees began trying to return to the Negev (Southern Israel), and there were no clear orders" (quoted in Magen 1991, p. 176).

As noted earlier, events of this kind intensify the soldier's emotional distress and deplete the resources for coping. When conditions already produce ethical conflicts, unclear orders add to the soldier's frustration, anger, confusion, and sense of powerlessness and lack of control. When the soldier, in such a complex situation, is left to interpret instructions for himself, his faith that his commanders will always be there to support him is undermined. Further complicating the ethical struggles of the soldier is the impact of public controversy over military actions. In a divided society, part of the public expects the soldier to use greater force and part abhors his actions, viewing them as aggressive, harmful, and inconsistent with human rights.

All of these things are known risk factors for the development of CSR. However, because Israeli society has trouble confronting the possibility of IDF involvement in actions of dubious legitimacy, soldiers' testimonies about such actions are often dismissed out of hand, and their trauma, caused by these actions, denied.

Five years after the outbreak of the First Lebanon War, the issue of purity of arms reemerged prominently within the IDF and Israeli public discourse. In late 1987, with the IDF still deep inside Lebanon, a popular uprising arose in the territories beyond the Green Line (the pre-1967 borders) unlike anything Israel had seen before.[14] Its participants included children and teenagers, and the entire Palestinian population came under suspicion of trying to harm Israeli soldiers and civilians. The military response to the uprising was forceful, and the new measures employed by the IDF led to an increase in inappropriate conduct on the part of soldiers. The army's activity was seen by the Israeli public as disproportionate, and even within the IDF there were those who objected to the violence perpetrated against a civilian population (Charlie Greenbaum, a senior reservist psychologist with the IDF's Behavioral Sciences Dept., quoted in Avissar n.d.).[15] The press was inundated by public criticism, which, if it did not necessarily reflect the position of the Israeli public as a whole, nevertheless expressed an attitude prevalent among broad swathes of the population, who, during the early stages at least, protested vociferously in the media, through petitions and at conferences (Peri 1990).[16]

The First Intifada (1987–1993) raised awareness about the dilemmas of the occupation and the harm inflicted on Palestinian civilians, but also drew attention to the possibility of psychological and moral harm to IDF soldiers serving in the territories.[17] Many commentators publicly expressed fears over the harmful effects of the soldiers' conflict when faced with the discrepancy between *jus ad bellum* and *jus in bello*. Experts in the field stressed that "soldiers have to be convinced not only that they are fighting for just goals, but also that, so far as possible, they are employing moral means to achieve those goals" (Hobfall & Milgram 1986, quoted in Gal 1990, p. 139).[18] Soldiers serving in the territories during the Intifada worked under a constant fear of being harmed, yet enjoyed blanket authorization to take violent measures when deemed necessary. Studies had already shown that such conditions could elicit violent behavior from people who in other situations would not act that way, or reinforce an already-present tendency toward violence (Gal 1990).[19] Indeed, commanders and mental health officers within the IDF began warning of psychological and moral damage to soldiers. In an explanatory letter written by IDF chief education officer Nehemia Dagan and disseminated to officers, he noted that the actions the IDF had found itself involved with during the Intifada "stand in the soldier's consciousness as something entirely different from the goals for whose sake he was conscripted" (Avissar 2007, p. 29). With time, however, commanders in the field admitted that soldiers got used to beating even though they were shocked by this policy. A Nahal (acronym of Noar Halutzi Lohem, lit. Fighting Pioneer Youth) battalion commander, who had participated in beating demonstrators with clubs, remarked, "The hardest thing? I think it's the meeting of the eyes. That second before the club falls on the demonstrator, when your eyes meet his. That physical proximity is disturbing, difficult. For many soldiers here it's a trauma, a personal trauma" (Emmanuel Rosen in Israeli daily *Maariv*, quoting Yisrael, commander of Nahal Airborne battalion; entire passage quoted by Avissar 2007, pp. 29–30).

The warnings and outcries from those active on the ground appear also to have influenced IDF chief of staff Dan Shomron, who asked two senior reservist psychologists to prepare a classified report on the functional status of soldiers in the Intifada and on the psychological ramifications of serving in the territories.[20] The report, which pointed to a deterioration of soldiers' restraint mechanisms, psychological damage, and a rise in the incidence of nightmares and depression, was dismissed by the IDF. Senior commanders prevented access of the report's authors to the chief of staff, who had commissioned it, or even to the head of the IDF's Manpower Directorate. At a later point the two psychologists were accused of leaking portions of the report to the press and were dismissed from their reserve posts (Avissar 2007).[21] Other attempts by civilian and military psychologists to call attention to the psychological and moral danger facing IDF soldiers met with similar reactions. Those who did express themselves publicly were accused of undermining IDF morale, of harboring the unrealistic expectation that military decisions be subject to the approval of "expert psychologists," and even of politicizing their professional activity (Ze'ev Schiff's article in the leading daily *Haaretz*, 1989, quoted in Dolev 1990). Military psychologists felt themselves torn between their allegiance to the individual soldier and to the system they were meant to represent.

Whether due to the personal price paid by critics, the accusations of disloyalty, or Israeli society's fear of its own reflection in the mirror, the critical voices ultimately died down, and the Israeli majority aligned itself with the security establishment's position. The senior officers in the IDF soon declared that the concerns that combat duty in the territories might have had a negative moral impact on soldiers had been unfounded, and the military denied any psychological impact from serving in the territories.[22]

A clear picture of the military-medical administration's denial of the psychological distress suffered by Israeli soldiers in the First Intifada can be gleaned from a series of interviews conducted by psychologist Nissim Avissar with the heads of the IDF's Mental Health Department and with senior psychologists serving in the field. Avissar found that "the army's mental health personnel both knew and didn't know . . . They sent out teams and held discussions, but at the same time they couldn't grasp—and in fact ignored—the information available to them" (Avissar n.d.; interviews from Avissar 2007). The Mental Health Department's official position, one subsequently shared by the state comptroller, reflected a similar conclusion regarding the absence of emotional distress: "There is no evidence . . . of psychological morbidity among soldiers due to IDF activity against the uprising in Judea, Samaria and the Gaza Strip." This conclusion, set forth in a state comptroller report on the IDF's handling of moral and psychological hazards to soldiers serving in the territories, was based on "the low number of soldier visits to mental health officers or mental health clinics, and on . . . the nature of these visits" (State Comptroller, Annual Report No. 40, quoted in Avissar 2007, p. 51).

So sweeping a denial of the Intifada's psychological fallout, and so resolute a disregard of the many firsthand testimonies available, may seem inexplicable given the progress made by the IDF since the establishment of the CSR Unit.[23] This denial, however, becomes comprehensible considering the political character of attitudes toward trauma in general, and toward trauma caused by controversial events in particular. In order to recognize CSR as the outcome of personal moral conflict experienced by soldiers carrying out IDF policy in the territories, there would have had to be a strict accounting of the effects of the Occupation and an attempt to answer the question that no one wanted to ask: Is the IDF still the world's most ethical army? Such recognition of CSR would also have cast doubt on the IDF's ability to maintain its routine activity in the conflict with the Palestinians, a conflict that most viewed as intractable.

In the face of such denial, the soldiers remained alone, which may well explain why so few of them sought assistance from the army's mental health services. Confronted with moral dilemmas on a day-to-day basis, the soldiers sought ways of mitigating the cognitive dissonance between the values according to which they felt they had been conscripted and the activities they found themselves performing. They had to build a wall between thought and feeling:

> I only remember that it's not okay. I don't believe in it. We stop the people . . . Or we beat them and a soldier stops someone and he says: "Leave me alone, I'm okay," so he punches him in the face. The first week it shocked me and I'd argue with people all the time, but after a while . . . you just remember that it's not okay, but you feel nothing.
>
> (Remarks of a soldier named Yoel, quoted by Liebes & Blum-Kulka 1990, p. 102)[24]

A few years after the First Intifada ended, and less than half a decade after the wave of terror attacks by Palestinian extremists who opposed the Oslo Accords had abated, the Second Intifada, or the Al-Aqsa Intifada, broke out (2000). The Second Intifada's impact on Israeli society and the widespread harm it caused to Israeli civilians will be taken up in Part II of this book. One issue that is not discussed there is the aforementioned societal difficulty—one that did not lessen over the years—of coping with moral injury, war trauma suffered by the inflictor of harm. A soldier who testified about the existence of this problem to the soldiers' organization "Breaking the Silence" called it transparent trauma due to society's denial of it (Sharon 2005). Public attitudes toward this issue during the Second Intifada are reflected in an article published by Professor Avi Bleich (2005), chair of the steering committee of Israel's Trauma Center for Victims of Terror and War (NATAL). Bleich's article presents NATAL's indecision over "whether it is appropriate to contact demobilized soldiers and offer them discussion and treatment for the psychological traumas that they endure in the wake of their military service." To the question of why an organization that cares for war trauma sufferers would hesitate on such an issue, the author answers that "there is a concern that discussion of the distress and trauma suffered by soldiers during the period of their service [in the territories], and particularly during the Intifada, might raise moral and ethical issues that would be automatically linked to political contexts and intentions that we, as professionals, wish to avoid association with" (Bleich 2005). In other words, Israeli society views trauma resulting from controversial military activity as a political issue, and therefore therapists who fear being labeled as politically motivated rather than objective and scientific hesitate to offer assistance to soldiers who have been traumatized in this way. This tendency to deny the existence of psychological trauma forced an organization like NATAL, devoted entirely to aiding trauma sufferers, into a political, rather than a therapeutic, quandary. Despite these concerns, NATAL ultimately decided, after lengthy internal deliberation, to stand behind the veterans and invite them to seek assistance.[25] A few years later, the organization held public screenings of films documenting psychological trauma resulting from serving in the second Intifada. However, discussions of the topic continue to be sensitive in NATAL, whose indecision reflects the tension that continues to surround the issue. Much of the Israeli public still reacts angrily when soldiers offer public testimonies on their traumatic confrontation with moral conflicts while fighting in a civilian area. The Israeli public interprets all such testimonies as political statements that undermine the IDF.[26] This approach also characterizes the IDF's CSR Unit. In a conversation with the author, the unit's commander at the time of writing this book persistently avoided questions about the attitude of the IDF to soldiers who developed PTSD due to routine operations amid the Palestinian population by asserting that it happened to only a small percentage of soldiers.[27] By contrast, Bleich et al. (2008) found a high percentage of exposure to traumatic events among soldiers who had served under such conditions. Over a third of the soldiers in the study's sample affirmed exposure to traumatic events in which they themselves had been the parties inflicting damage, and 17% of these soldiers regarded their actions as having humiliated the Palestinians, a view that is known as a risk factor for developing trauma due to the inner conflict that it creates.

Opposition to confronting the trauma experienced by soldiers who have injured civilians is found not only among those who deny the possibility of IDF soldiers being involved in such inappropriate acts. Some take the opposite position, similar to Allan Young, contending that soldiers are directly responsible for their own actions and therefore do not merit the empathy that trauma deserves. As these critics see it, soldier testimonies of suffering while witnessing or even participating in misdeeds during combat constitute a "rite of passage" that enables soldiers to "prove they have a conscience" and to evade responsibility for their actions. Rather than refusing to take part in such acts and paying the price, these critics say, through the public testimonials soldiers "absolve themselves" of any blame and then return to their military service (Elgazi 2004).

When discussing these issues it is important to take into account the great differences between the Vietnam War and the situation in Israel. Atrocities such as those committed in My Lai and other Vietnamese villages are unheard of in Israel. For one thing, combat conditions in Vietnam were much harsher than those encountered by IDF soldiers, where the physical distance between Vietnam and the US cut the American soldiers off from their homes and support networks, thereby impairing their psychological resilience and clouding their moral judgment. Despite these differences, one finds similarities between the two situations on the question of moral responsibility and the personal and social significance of recognizing trauma caused to soldiers by harming civilians, sometimes intentionally but many times unintentionally. Similarities also exist with regard to the inner conflict that takes place in the souls of many soldiers during military operations amid a civilian population.

The situations discussed earlier produced a new category of war trauma: "moral injury," which only recently has begun to draw researchers' attention (Litz et al. 2009; Dokoupil 2012; Keynan 2013).[28] This term addresses the trauma caused in morally ambiguous conditions created by the new nature of war within civilian areas. The testimony of American soldiers who have served in Iraq and Afghanistan, like that of Israeli soldiers who have served in Gaza, Lebanon, and the West Bank, shows that the new nature of war undermines the often-used term "self-traumatized perpetrator." This term is disputed in the US, and in Israel it is interpreted as an attempt to tarnish the IDF and smear its soldiers. I believe that this blame term should be used only to describe incidents of extreme and intentional violence, whose participants should indeed bear sole responsibility for their resulting trauma. The term "self-traumatized perpetrator" is too wide, and isolates all soldiers as the guilty parties, tending to free both state and society from any responsibility for the soldiers' fate or the conditions that gave rise to the controversial acts in the first place.

The expression "moral injury," on the other hand, reflects the difficulties faced by soldiers in morally ambiguous and stressful situations, and it also emphasizes the fact that wars induce suffering among innocent civilians as well as those defined as enemies. Therefore, in contrast to the former, it does not free societies and governments from their moral responsibility.

In a way, the opposition to recognizing the trauma suffered by those who are agents of violence is the new form of CSR denial. In Israel, the taboo against even discussing the phenomenon is reminiscent of the forbidden pain of battle-shock sufferers during the early decades of Israeli statehood. Whether a response to the threat of delegitimizing Israel's cause in its conflict with the Palestinians, or whether out of a desire to highlight the unjust occupation, the taboo from both sides of the political debate leaves traumatized soldiers isolated in their suffering. In many cases they are unable to share their feelings even with their fellow soldiers for fear of being regarded as traitors for openly discussing things best kept quiet.[29] While any intentional harm perpetrated by soldiers upon civilians, or any indifference to such acts, must be unequivocally denounced, one should not deny or obscure the plight of soldiers who, against their will, find themselves in a pernicious reality that entails harm to innocents, or, in Lifton's words, "atrocity producing situations."

Over the last few years, films have played a role in raising public awareness of the trauma suffered by soldiers subsequent to acts they themselves took part in: *Waltz with Bashir* (2008), *Lebanon* (2009), and *Shurot Shurot* (2008).[30] These films, particularly *Waltz with Bashir*, reflect the convoluted nature of the Israeli-Palestinian conflict and shed light on the complex issue of responsibility within that conflict. The films also point up the elusive and delayed character of psychological trauma, thereby raising the possibility that the number of those afflicted with moral injury is much greater than generally acknowledged. Israeli society would do well to undertake a thorough moral accounting of the nature of its war with the Palestinians. Regardless of whether it does so, it should relinquish its latest form of PTSD denial. Traumatized IDF soldiers afflicted with moral injury are left to suffer alone, while Israeli society conveys mixed messages and ignores the personal price that these soldiers pay for its decisions. Even after demobilization, the soldiers live with a sense of distress and solitude. They struggle with forbidden feelings and a suppressed moral conflict, a conflict that no one who has experienced can put behind him:

> The army doesn't tell you during basic training that you're going to be living with it for the rest of your life. The army doesn't tell you about everything you're going to go through afterward . . . About fellow soldiers who wet their beds in the army, about friends of mine who aren't finding themselves, who nearly two years after demobilization are lying on the couch and don't know what to do with their lives.
>
> (Paratrooper who traveled to India for a prolonged period, quoted in Sharon 2005)

Notes

This work does not aim to address the Israeli-Arab conflict from a moral or political perspective. The analysis offered here focuses solely on the ramifications of the change in the characteristics of warfare over the last few decades, on the domestic Israeli debate regarding the scope of traumatic injury to soldiers, and on the societal processes by which such injury is denied or acknowledged.

1. The citation "war of choice" is from *Maariv* (20 August 1982). Quoted statement of then prime minister Menachem Begin.

2. "They [the bereaved parents] harbor the terrible suspicion that the sacrifice was not unavoidable," wrote Mordechai Shmuel, a bereaved father, in an article published in *Maariv* on 11 July 1974, entitled, "Bereaved Parents: We Don't Feel the Public Is Sensitive to Our Plight," quoted by Lebel (2008).
3. "I'm telling you, son, it was an unnecessary war," as Alex L., a bereaved father, put it in a poem (in Hever & Ron 2006, p. 38).
4. Y. Smilansky, 1985, "At the Foot of the Monument to Our Fallen in Israel's Wars" [Speech at the unveiling of the memorial site honoring Tel Aviv University's war casualties, Tel Aviv University], 7 November.
5. The Occupied Territories refer to the territories conquered by Israel in 1967, in the West Bank (also known as Judea and Samaria) and before 2005 also the Gaza strip, from which Israel withdrew in that year.
6. For protest songs, see "Come Here Airplane Flying By, Take Us Up into the Sky, Sharon Will Send Us to Attack, in a Coffin We'll Come Back." The soldiers were filmed by television reporter Dan Semama for a story that set off a political storm in 1984 (Kam 2009). Some 170 had refused to serve by 1980, according to Gal (1990).
7. This anthology of anti-war poems was commissioned jointly by Sifriat Poalim and a group of bereaved parents whose sons had fallen in the Battle of the Beaufort.
8. Of those recognized as PTSD sufferers, 43.5% were injured in the Yom Kippur War, and 42.3% in the First Lebanon War. Presentation of Professor Yossi Zohar before the Goren Committee (see chapter 4), slide 8. From the time the war broke out until the IDF withdrew from Lebanon 1,216 soldiers were killed. During the war itself 620 of them fell in the summer of 1982. Rubenstein (2008, p. 234) cites data presented by Zahava Solomon in a 1984 follow-up study by the IDF Mental Health Department, according to which 493 CSR sufferers had been treated by the Department as of February 1983. That figure does not reflect the sum total of the psychologically wounded, but merely the number of those who had sought treatment up to that time. It constitutes a very high proportion of the total number of those wounded during the first nine months of the war.
9. Term borrowed from Sharon (2005).
10. See the asterisked note to Chapter 1.
11. On 16 March 1968, soldiers of a US Army battalion slaughtered, in cold blood and with no provocation, hundreds of inhabitants of the Vietnamese village of My Lai, most of them women, children, babies, and elderly people. Estimates of the number of killings range from 347 to 504. Many of the villagers were tortured and subjected to sexual abuse before being killed; soldiers even mutilated their bodies. A helicopter pilot from a different unit and two of his crewmembers tried to protect the villagers, threatening to fire on soldiers who shot at the Vietnamese. They managed to rescue only ten villagers, whom they flew to safety in their helicopter; the pilot having reported the incident to his superior officers, the slaughter was finally halted. The My Lai massacre was an incident of critical importance in the Vietnam War, one that intensified protest activity both in the US and abroad.
12. Per Israeli Penal Law, 5737–1977, Clause 34 M: "No person shall bear criminal responsibility for an act, which he committed [. . .] under the order of a competent authority, which he was obligated to obey under Law, unless the order was obviously unlawful." Per Clause 20 of the Military Justice Law, 5715–1955, "The soldier is justified if the act which he committed, which constitutes an offense, was committed [. . .] in order to avoid, during the execution of a military mission, refusal to obey a lawful command issued for the purposes of that mission, or non-compliance with such a command." The law restricts the justification defense by making it applicable only in instances where there was no other way to avoid refusal to obey or noncompliance with the order, and only if the soldier did not "go beyond what was necessary for that purpose." Compliance with a manifestly unlawful order does not constitute a defense.

13. On the vagueness of orders and directives and its impact on soldiers during the First Intifada, see statement of Joel Elitzur, a reservist psychologist with the IDF mental health services, quoted in Avissar (2007). On strategies for coping with the dissonance, see Liebes and Blum-Kulka (1990).
14. This was the beginning of the First Intifada that lasted until 1991.
15. Greenbaum's statement is taken from a set of interviews that Avissar conducted in the framework of his doctoral dissertation with psychologists who had served in the IDF during the First Intifada (see Avissar 2007).
16. For examples of public criticism in the press, see Avissar (2007), pp. 29–31.
17. On aspects of the First Intifada's impact on Israeli society, see Gal (1990).
18. Gal himself, as we shall see ahead, dismissed concerns over psychological and moral harm to IDF soldiers.
19. Gal mentions Philip Zimbardo's well-known prison experiment (1972) and Stanley Milgram's equally famous electric shock experiment from the 1960s. See also Bleich et al. (2008); Zimbardo (2004).
20. Professor Charlie Greenbaum, chief psychologist of the Central Command, and Professor Dan Bar-On, chief psychologist of the Southern Command.
21. The two psychologists denied having leaked data to the press, but stood behind the general assessments that they voiced in media interviews after they had despaired of presenting their findings to the chief of staff or to other senior figures in the IDF high command.
22. Gal (1990, p. 138) writes, "This fear of 'pathological damage' and 'a heavy psychological price' was found to be exaggerated and unsubstantiated." The article is, in essence, a lecture that Gal delivered at a 1988 conference devoted to the issue. Colonel (Res.) Reuven Gal served as the IDF's chief psychologist prior to the outbreak of the Intifada and held a variety of other psychology-related posts within the military.
23. See, for example, the soldier interviews in Liebes and Blum-Kulka (1990) and the classified psychologists' report.
24. See also Liebes and Blum-Kulka's (1990) discussion of soldiers' sense of dissonance and indecision.
25. Author's conversation with the NATAL Steering Committee on 11 January 2010. Statement of Avi Bleich.
26. See reactions to the Israeli film *Waltz with Bashir* (2008), which highlights the traumatic experiences of a soldier in the First Lebanon War. Although the film was celebrated for its cinematic quality, many accused it of being "anti-Israeli." See the following talkbacks (retrieved on 8 January 2010): www.ynet.co.il/Ext/App/TalkBack/CdaView OpenTalkBack/0,11382,L-3631548,00.html. Soldiers involved in the organization Breaking the Silence also encounter considerable hostility, including attempts by the establishment to prevent the organization from receiving donations from abroad. ('Don't Silence Breaking the Silence' 2009).
27. Levy interview, 2009.
28. Moral injury can also occur as a result of feeling guilt for the death of comrades, but this kind of war trauma is not disputed.
29. On the fear of other soldiers in one's unit, see *To See if I'm Smiling* (2007); also, the Breaking the Silence website: www.shovrimshtika.org .
30. See Ari Folman (director) (2008), *Waltz with Bashir* (film, Israel); Shmuel Maoz (director) (2009), *Lebanon* (film, Israel); *To See if I'm Smiling* (2007). See also Netiva Ben-Yehuda's remarks in the documentary film *Shurot Shurot* (2008). Ben-Yehuda describes the memories and events that continue to haunt her since the War of Independence, including friends who were killed "and also [pause] those whom you killed." After the phrase "and also" she becomes silent, absorbed in lighting her cigarette; the remainder of the sentence is uttered in a low voice, one that has trouble both saying and not saying.

References

American Psychiatric Association 1980, *Diagnostic and Statistical Manual of Mental Disorders*, 3rd edn., Washington D.C.

Avissar, N. 2007, *Psychology, Social Responsibility and Political Involvement: the First Intifada and Israeli Psychologists*, doctoral dissertation, Bar-Ilan University. (Hebrew)

Avissar, N. (n.d.), 'A Close Look at Blurring, Denial and Silencing: the Army Psychologists and the First Intifada' in *Psychoactive—Mental Health Professionals for Human Rights*. Available from www.psychoactive.org.il [3 January 2009].

Bleich, A. 2005, 'The Distress Suffered by Demobilized Soldiers: Should It Be Placed on the Public Agenda?', *B'Nogea L'Regesh*, vol. 7. Available from www.natal.org.il/?CategoryID=327&ArticleID=267 [8 January 2010]. (Hebrew)

Bleich, A., Gelkopf, M., Berger, R., & Solomon, Z. 2008, 'The Psychological Toll of the Intifada: Symptoms of Distress and Coping in Israeli Soldiers', *IMAJ*, vol. 10, pp. 873–876. (Hebrew)

Cook, M. L. 2001, 'Ethical Issues in War: an Overview' in *U.S. Army War College Guide to Strategy*, eds. J. R. Cerami & J. F. Holcomb, Strategic Studies Institute, Derby, PA, pp. 19–30.

Dokoupil, T. 2012, 'A New Theory of PTSD and Veterans: Moral Injury', *Newsweek*, 12 December.

Dolev, A. 1990, 'Psychologists Involvement in Actual Events – the Issue of Professional Neutrality'. In *The Seventh War: the Effects of the Intifada on Israeli Society*, ed. R. Gal, Hakibbutz Hameuchad, Tel Aviv, pp. 149–155. (Hebrew)

'Don't Silence Breaking the Silence' 2009. Available from www.btselem.org/Hebrew/Press_Releases/20090802.asp [2 August 2009].

Elgazi, G. 2004, 'Listen to the Voice of Refusal' in *The Refusnik Trials*, eds. D. Khenin, M. Sfard, & S. Rothbard, Babel, Tel Aviv, pp. 11–35.

Gal, R. 1990, 'Psychological and Moral Aspects of the IDF Soldiers' Experience with the Intifada' in *The Seventh War: the Effects of the Intifada on Israeli Society*, ed. R. Gal, Hakibbutz Hameuchad, Tel Aviv, pp. 135–148. (Hebrew)

Hever, H., & Ron, M. (eds.) 2006, *Fighting and Killing without End: Poems of the Lebanon War* (revised edition), Hakibbutz Hameuchad, Tel Aviv.

Kam, A. 2009, 'Journalist Dan Semama Dies', *Walla (!) News*, 22 February.

Kashti, Y., & Rimon Or, A. 1999, 'Security, Identity and Education', in *Modernity, Post-Modernity, and Education*, ed. I. Gur-Ze'ev, Ramot, Ra'anana, pp. 165–196. (Hebrew)

Keynan, I. 2013, 'Moral Injury and Moral Responsibility: the Case of Israel'. Paper presented at the 21th Annual UC Interdisciplinary Psychoanalytic Consortium, Lake Arrowhead Conference Center. Los Angeles, California.

Lebanon 2009, motion picture.

Lebel, U. 2008, 'Cracks in the Hegemonic Bereavement Model: the Political Behavior of the Families of Soldiers Killed in the Yom Kippur War' in *National Trauma: the Yom Kippur War: a Retrospective of Thirty Years and Another War*, eds. M. Shemesh & Z. Drori, Ben-Gurion Institute and Ben-Gurion University, Sde Boker, pp. 325–349.

Liebes, T., & Blum-Kulka, S. 1990, 'Shooting and Crying? On Confronting Moral Dilemmas during Intifada Military Service', in *The Seventh War: the Effects of the Intifada on Israeli Society*, ed. R. Gal, Hakibbutz Hameuchad, Tel Aviv, pp. 85–106. (Hebrew)

Lifton, R. J. 2005, *Home from the War*, Other Press, New York.

Litz, B. T., Stein, N., Delaney, E., Lebowitz, L., Nash, W. P., Silva, C., & Maguen, S. 2009, 'Moral Injury and Moral Repair in War Veterans: a Preliminary Model and Intervention Strategy', *Clinical Psychology*, vol. 29, pp. 695–706.

Magen, A. (ed.) 1991, *Purity of Arms*, Yad Tabenkin and the Israel Society for Military History in association with Tel Aviv University, Ramat Efal.

Megged, A. 1982, 'Ethics in Wartime', *Davar*, 18 June.

Military Prosecutor v. Major Malinki et al. 1957, Military Court, MR 3/57. (Hebrew)

Neria, Y., Solomon, Z., Ginsberg, K., Dekel, R., Enoch, D., & Ohry, A. 1998, 'Wars and Their Psychological Cost: Aspects of Psychological Trauma among Soldiers and Civilians in Israeli Society', *Society and Welfare*, vol. 18, no. 1, pp. 125–139. (Hebrew)

Oz, A. 1982, 'Where Shall We Hide the Shame', *Davar*, 22 June.

Peri, Y. 1990, 'The Intifada's Impact on the IDF', in *The Seventh War: the Effects of the Intifada on Israeli Society*, ed. R. Gal, Hakibbutz Hameuchad, Tel Aviv, pp. 122–128. (Hebrew)

Rubenstein, Z. 2008, *From Battle Shock to Combat Stress Reaction: a History of Paradigm Change in the Yom Kippur and Lebanon Wars, as Reflected in the Care-Provider and Mental Health Systems Narrative*, doctoral dissertation, Tel Aviv University. (Hebrew)

Scott, W. J. 1990, 'PTSD in DSM-III: a Case in the Politics of Diagnosis and Disease', *Social Problems*, vol. 37, no. 3, pp. 294–310.

Sharon A. 2005, 'Transparent Trauma', *Breaking the Silence*. Available from www.shovrimshtika.org/article.asp?id=5&page=2 [7 July 2009].

Shurot Shurot 2008, documentary film.

Sidon, E. 1983, 'Children' in *Border Crossing: Poems of the Lebanon War*, ed. J. Kafri, Sifriat Poalim, Tel Aviv, p. 39. (Hebrew)

Smilansky, Y. 1985, *At the Foot of the Monument to Our Fallen in Israel's Wars* [Speech at the unveiling of the memorial site honoring Tel Aviv University's war casualties, Tel Aviv University], 7 September.

To See if I'm Smiling 2007, documentary film.

Waltz with Bashir 2008, motion picture.

Young, A. 2002, 'The Self-Traumatized Perpetrator as a "Transient Mental Illness"', *L'Évolution Psychiatrique*, vol. 67, pp. 630–650.

Zimbardo, P. G. 2004, 'A Situationist Perspective on the Psychology of Evil: Understanding How Good People Are Transformed into Perpetrators', in *The Social Psychology of Good and Evil*, ed. A. Miller, Guilford, New York, pp. 21–50.

6 Combat Stress Reaction in an Era of Social Privatization

The soldiers' belief that they are part of a larger military apparatus capable of ensuring their safety, their confidence in the loyalty of their comrades and commanders, and their faith in the support of the society that sent them into battle are three of the most prominent factors that studies have identified as protecting soldiers against CSR. But over the past decade, the Israeli public's faith in the state's commitment to its soldiers has eroded. This erosion, fueled by growing criticism of the army, a rising awareness of the disintegration of social solidarity, and growing economic privatization and social fragmentation, has produced a crisis of values that increases the risk of CSR.

These processes emerged during the last quarter of the twentieth century concomitant with social and intellectual transformations then appearing in Israel. The strong commitment to the collective that had previously characterized Israeli society began to give way to concern for the needs and rights of the individual, and Israeli collective identity began to show fissures that reflected major social rifts. Israel's social heterogeneity increased significantly with the arrival of some 70,000 new immigrants from Ethiopia (since 1977) and a million from the former Soviet Union (since 1989), and with the increasing stridency with which groups such as the "Mizrahim" (Jewish immigrants from the Islamic countries) demanded economic equality and recognition of their identity and culture (Yonah 2005). The success of neoliberal ideas led to increased privatization, which, against a background of rapid globalization, deepened socioeconomic gaps, weakened existing social programs, and undermined values of mutual commitment.

At the same time, a new postmodern skepticism toward "grand narratives" began to take root and the notion of singular Jewish-Israeli identity disintegrated (Lyotard 1979). The myths that held sway during the early decades of Israeli statehood began to erode, replaced by a multiplicity of narratives, at times in conflict with each other. Fundamental beliefs were shaken by new theories critical of nationalism in general, and of Israeli nationalism in particular. During the 1990s an ongoing dispute over Zionism's beginnings burst the confines of the ivory tower, and the analyses put forward by the "New Historians" fueled bitter disagreements about the past and about the present. These controversies over the history of the State of Israel, erupting during an era of skepticism about national myths, cultivated a post-Zionist perspective among a portion of the Israeli public.

This controversy merged with an already-vitiated sense of absolute Israeli justice in the conflict with the Palestinians, extending the doubts to debates over the responsibility for the creation of the Palestinian refugees in the War of Independence (Morris 1989).

Despite these changes, basic popular assumptions regarding the Israeli-Palestinian conflict have remained unchanged. Most Israelis continue to believe that the State of Israel exists under constant threat, regardless of its actions, and that the Israeli-Palestinian conflict is intractable. Israeli society is characterized by a siege mentality, which, according to Daniel Bar-Tal, causes a large portion of the public to view the rest of the world as sinister in its intentions toward Israel (Bar-Tal 2007). Life in the shadow of such beliefs is especially difficult for a divided and factious society in which any security-related or political action sets off stormy debates. The contradiction between beliefs in the intractability of national conflict and doubts regarding the justice of the cause makes for an absurd situation: there are widespread expectations of inevitable war without end alongside doubts over the necessity of the wars and how they should be conducted.

Amid these controversies and doubts yet another time-honored consensus—the belief that the IDF should be sheltered from any controversy, internal or external—has collapsed, and along with it the myths linked to that consensus. The IDF still enjoys a high degree of public favor and support, but these feelings have weakened considerably as elements of ambivalence have permeated the public discourse.[1] Although most Israelis feel dependent on the IDF and regard its soldiers as "everybody's sons," the army has nevertheless become subject to criticism and condemnation. Attempts to keep the separation between the affection for soldiers and criticism of the senior defense leadership have failed time and again. The IDF no longer enjoys the shielding it once did from public scrutiny or the expression of doubt.

Maintaining the IDF's legitimacy has become even harder given its involvement in national controversies, such as the evacuation of Israeli citizens from settlements, when the army is forced to clash with those it is normally enjoined to defend. Such situations blur the distinction between a protected and sympathetic population and a critical, hostile population. I will not enter here into a discussion of the complex relationship between the IDF and the residents of the settlements. It is, however, crucial to note that the need to use force against Jewish citizens of Israel and the antagonistic behavior with which these citizens greet the army and every soldier who takes part in evacuation operations—shouting, spitting, cursing, and, at times, physical violence—give rise to a confusing and distressing atmosphere that creates an additional risk factor for trauma.[2]

One conspicuous indication of the sea of change that has occurred both in the relations between the army and society and in the value systems espoused by Israelis can be seen in the way that individuals deal with bereavement. The reaction to bereavement has become more private and personal, reflecting a new perspective that sees the soldier as belonging first and foremost to his family (Rosenthal 2001). In accordance with this perspective, bereaved families now demand that they be allowed to commemorate their loved ones privately, rather than in a collective manner dictated by the state. They seek a full account of the actions where their sons fell, even when such information might cause them great pain. Nor do they flinch from vehemently and publicly criticizing the Israeli security forces at all levels.[3] On the other hand, as we shall see ahead, the change in values is also reflected in the way that the IDF and the state perceive their commitment to the personal fate of each soldier.

Doubts about the degree of the state's commitment to IDF soldiers stem firstly from the public sense that, during the first decade of the twenty-first century, there has been an erosion among the political and military leadership of the deep-seated Israeli principle that no solider should ever be left behind. This principle, which at times necessitates difficult choices between sometimes contradictory values—for example, putting at risk the lives of soldiers in order to rescue a wounded soldier—is a major factor in the prevention of CSR. This is not to claim that in the past units never abandoned a wounded soldier on the battlefield or that the state was never neglectful in its efforts to bring home POWs and soldiers missing in action. But until a decade ago, the public regarded such instances as one-time failures, whereas now it views them as the product of a fundamental systemic change.

In the following pages I will briefly analyze three events that conspicuously illustrate this development: the death of IDF soldier Madhat Yusuf, the failures to evacuate wounded soldiers during the Second Lebanon War, and the controversy over the agreement to secure the release of Gilad Shalit.

The first indication of the erosion of the principle of leaving no one behind came on October 10, 2001, the second day of the El-Aqsa Intifada, with the death of IDF serviceman Madhat Yusuf, a Border Police corporal, serving in Nablus and stationed with 11 other soldiers at Joseph's Tomb, a small isolated shrine. Yusuf sustained a bullet wound to the neck when 100 or so armed Palestinians attacked the shrine compound, surrounding it. While his fellow soldiers tried to treat his wounds, the severity of the injury required his transfer to a hospital. Based on the calculation that evacuating Yusuf by force might end in a bloodbath for both sides, Prime Minister Ehud Barak instructed Chief of Staff Shaul Mofaz to refrain from military action to evacuate the wounded soldier and instead to negotiate his evacuation with Jibril Rajoub, head of the Palestinian Authority's Preventive Security Force. Rajoub repeatedly postponed his arrival at the scene of the incident and ultimately did nothing to aid Yusuf's evacuation. Despite repeated pleas by the medic and commanders stationed at the compound, who watched as Yusuf bled to death, the Israeli security leadership adhered to their decision not to evacuate Yusuf by force. The fact that an injured serviceman had been left to die in the field, with the full knowledge of the prime minister and the IDF's most senior commanders, aroused consternation both within and outside the IDF, particularly in light of the conscious decision on which the abandonment was based—a decision that was never denied and that is actually documented on the memorial website to fallen Israeli soldiers maintained by the Defense Ministry.[4] Chief Education Officer Elazar Stern dismissed the criticism, arguing that the value of evacuating a single wounded soldier had been weighed carefully against the necessity of putting many soldiers at risk in a rescue effort (IDF Manpower

Directorate, 2000). Stern even added that the IDF had never adhered to a norm of evacuating wounded soldiers under all conditions and at all costs: "Disregarding the cost, as well as the conditions in the field, constitutes a misunderstanding of the nature of command."[5] Many Israelis felt these statements, coming from the officer responsible for disseminating the values of the Israeli military, signaled a fundamental change in policy and attitude. Others saw the dispelling of an illusion under which they had long been laboring, but which perhaps had never reflected reality—an even more disturbing possibility. The incident caused public outrage and prompted demonstrations by reservists, who felt that a crossroads had been reached in the relations between soldiers and the senior military leadership.[6] This marked the start of a wrenching and impassioned public debate over the cost of rescuing a soldier and over the IDF's commitment to the value of not leaving wounded servicemen, POWs, and MIAs behind.[7]

The second indication that the value of nonabandonment was disintegrating came during the Second Lebanon War. Launched in July 2006, the war eroded public confidence in Israel's political and military leadership and left the country deeply polarized. Many felt that the war had been undertaken recklessly, military instructions issued during the fighting were vague and conflicting, and, in the end, the army failed to achieve a decisive victory or put an end to the firing of rockets on Israel from southern Lebanon.[8] Among the bitter and divisive questions raised by the war, the issue of the state's obligation to wounded soldiers and POWs took on particular significance. The immediate reason for the war was, purportedly, to rescue two Israeli soldiers, Eldad Regev and Ehud Goldwasser, who had been abducted by Hezbollah and whom the IDF believed to still be alive. The IDF's failure to extricate wounded soldiers during this war seems, with this mission in mind, like a bitter historical irony.

Soldiers who fought in the Second Lebanon War testify to a resurfacing of the image of Madhat Yusuf while they witnessed long delays in the evacuation of wounded servicemen, and to too many instances of soldiers left in the field, bleeding to death. "In this war I repressed Madhat Yusuf," said one reservist who participated in the Second Lebanon War. "I didn't think about it. When I saw the wounded soldiers . . . it came back to me . . . It's not a matter of fear, of 'Oh, no, I'll be left here alone, what's going to happen?' It's anger . . . that they can do something like that" (*May Every Mother Know* 2007). The testimonies indicate that many IDF soldiers linked these recent abandonments to the death of Madhat Yusuf, which they identified as the moment when the previously sacred norm began to unravel (ibid.; statement of Or Noy, tank crewmember). "Evacuating wounded soldiers isn't something you calculate in terms of chances and percentages. It has to be an absolute truth that when someone is wounded you evacuate him, whatever the risk . . . At the time the Madhat Yusuf incident happened, that was one of my greatest disillusionments with the army" (ibid.).

The soldiers' memory of the events at Joseph's Tomb was tinged with anger and frustration, which intensified with a growing awareness that the Yusuf incident reflected a new policy and a profound change in values. "In this war I learned a new term, 'delayed evacuation.' What does it mean? That you're left there at least until nightfall. You're wounded at eight in the morning. Now your evacuation is being delayed. A sterile kind of a word" (ibid.).

These claims are not substantiated by the report of the Commission of Inquiry into the Events of the 2006 Campaign (the Winograd Commission), established in response to intense public pressure to investigate the different aspects of the Second Lebanon War. The commission members viewed the decision by commanders in the field not to allow the evacuation of wounded soldiers during daylight hours as a reasonable one "given the assessment that great risk would be involved, both to the helicopters and to the injured servicemen."[9] However, it is precisely this approach that the soldiers, especially reservists who had served in previous wars, regard as indicative of a new norm to which they cannot reconcile themselves. They return again and again to the Joseph's Tomb incident, a repetitiveness that embodies an element of trauma, and ask whether that was the beginning of "this devaluation of human life" (*May Every Mother Know* 2007, statement of Gen. [Res.] Doron Rubin).

A significant number of Israeli soldiers suffered CSR and combat PTSD in the Second Lebanon War. In April 2008 the head of the Defense Ministry's Disabled Rehabilitation Division, Brigadier General Roni Moreno, announced an endeavor to identify CSR and combat PTSD sufferers from the Second Lebanon War, predicting that hundreds of not-yet-diagnosed soldiers suffered from post-traumatic symptoms, which, as is known, often emerge after considerable delay. As of July 2011 the Rehabilitation Division had classified 203 soldiers as PTSD sufferers with disability ratings of over 20% (the minimum level required to qualify for services from the Division), as compared with 17 soldiers in Operation Cast Lead.[10] The main reason for this high rate of trauma was the chaotic conditions under which the soldiers fought. Unclear goals about which no consensus existed and conflicting and inconsistent orders gave soldiers the feeling that they didn't "know where they [were] going or where they [were] headed," a major and well-known risk factor for the development of CSR.[11] The issue of the slow or reluctant evacuation of wounded soldiers certainly compounded rates of CSR. As noted earlier, trauma researchers discovered years ago that a soldier's faith in the military system's ability and willingness to come to his aid and defend him, even under the most trying conditions, is a central component of his illusion of safety, which constitutes an important defense against the occurrence of CSR. The absence of such faith increases the risk for CSR.

This issue also lies at the heart of public debate over the deal negotiated for the release of Gilad Shalit, a soldier abducted near the Kerem Shalom border crossing by a Hamas cell on June 25, 2006, 17 days prior to the eruption of the Second Lebanon War. The Hamas members killed two IDF soldiers in the raid and took the wounded Shalit to an unknown location in the Gaza Strip. For more than five years Israel was unable to reach an agreement that would result in the soldier's release. The demands posed by Hamas during negotiations fueled a new round of a familiar debate over the "price" that should or should not be "paid" for a soldier's return home, a question that divides Israeli society whenever soldiers are taken prisoner.[12] The debate aroused strong feelings both among those who supported reaching an agreement at virtually any price and among those who opposed releasing Palestinian prisoners "with blood on their hands" as part of an exchange. The entire discussion was haunted by the specter of captured pilot Ron Arad, who had been taken prisoner in Lebanon by the Amal organization in 1986. The negotiations for his release failed, all traces of him disappeared, and he remains missing to this day. The Ron Arad affair, which left Israeli society with a gaping wound, was a rare instance of failure to bring a POW home. Unlike the Madhat Yusuf incident, it was not at first perceived as a case of abandonment but rather as a failure. With the passing of time, however, criticism of how the government handled the Arad affair has intensified, and some have raised the question of whether enough was actually done.[13]

Those who supported negotiating a deal for Gilad Shalit's release viewed the commitment to soldiers as a supreme value and the willingness to pay a huge price in order to bring POWs home as an expression of a strong and determined society, undeterred by the enemy's gloating about its so called "good bargain" in exchange for just one soldier. For them it is both a clear agreement between Israeli society and its soldiers and critical for the IDF's strength. They called for the unwritten contract between the army and its soldiers to be upheld, and argued that the price of failing to bring a POW home would be higher than the cost of his release (Keynan 2008; Zakai 2009). Those opposed to the idea of striking a deal regarded the proposed agreement as an expression of weakness and of "capitulation" to the enemy, which would in turn lead to more abductions. They demanded unconditional sacrifice of the soldier and his family and emphasized that releasing prisoners who had been involved in terrorist attacks would endanger other Israelis, who might lose their lives in additional attacks. Amid these arguments, the position of General (Res.) Yaakov Amidror is of particular interest. In an appearance before the Shamgar Committee, tasked with setting principles for negotiating ransoms for redemption of POWs, in June 2009, he stated that despite his opposition in principle to negotiations for the return of abductees, "in the specific instance of Gilad Shalit, Israel has lost the moral right [to refrain from negotiating] and has violated its contract with the abducted soldier." He based his assertion on an overall approach dictating that abductees be evacuated by force, meaning that Operation Cast Lead should not have been terminated without bringing Gilad home (quoted in Bergman 2009, p. 578).[14] Amidror's stance appeared to support preserving the once-sacred norm of bringing soldiers home under any conditions. From his point of view, the disagreement concerned how to do it—by force or via negotiations.

An analysis of the opposing views regarding Gilad Shalit's release brings us back, once again, to the Madhat Yusuf affair. In a talk with high school students, Defense Minister Ehud Barak discussed the government's efforts to bring about Shalit's release. His appeal to "every young person in the country [not to] think in terms of whining or losing one's backbone" reflects his position that "combatants and soldiers are conscripted in the knowledge that fulfilling the mission entails preparedness to sacrifice one's life." This is the stance that found expression in his decision nine years earlier, as prime minister, not to evacuate Yusuf by force. In a discussion of Gilad Shalit, Barak deflected criticism of the government and said that despite "the moral and military responsibility to Gilad Shalit," he should not be brought back "at any price."[15] Once again we hear the echo of Chief Education Officer Elazar Stern's denial in 2000 of the existence of values that have to be upheld at all costs. These statements, coming from leaders of the defense establishment, reflect incongruity between the soldier's willingness to lay down his life and his expectation of a similar commitment on the part of the state, and they miss the point that this expectation does not stem from a weakened spirit of self-sacrifice, but rather the opposite. It is the state's weakened commitment that erodes the soldier's commitment to self-sacrifice and to placing the mission first.

These arguments over price generate another troubling dynamic in which the effort to gain a POW's release becomes the family's private endeavor. Such may be inferred from an analysis of the Shalit family's struggle and from the efforts of other families before them. The intention here is not to claim that the state has shirked its responsibility toward POWs, but to emphasize that the families, and many other citizens, have recognized that at least some of the prospects for the POW's return depend on their own efforts and on the pressure that they can exert on the government and other parties involved in the negotiations. This dynamic, which has repeated itself over the last few decades, further diminishes confidence in the state and the military. It raises questions about reciprocity and about how responsibility is divided between the state and the individual and gives rise to a sense that the state is unable to honor "its contract with the citizens."[16] In the past such disagreements were obscured, whether because censorship prevented the information from reaching the public at large or because the incidents were regarded as exceptions to the IDF's policy and standards. Once the messages from the security establishment changed, blatantly and officially, a Pandora's box opened, setting off an emotional tempest in the public sphere over one of the most basic features of Israel's national ethos.

This is not the place to assess the various perspectives on the topic. The aforementioned examples do, however, illustrate the depth, intensity, and painfulness of the dispute, which has tormented the IDF and Israeli society over the past decade. They reveal the dispute's ramifications for soldier morale on the battlefield and for the morale of families on the home front—one of which is an increased risk for CSR and combat PTSD.

Part III of the book will address claims recently made—from both within and outside of the military establishment—that the problem of war trauma in Israel has radically shifted from denial to exaggeration, so much so that the situation has gotten out of hand. Not only does our discussion in the present part refute these claims, but it also calls attention to new risk factors previously unknown in Israel. These risk factors are linked to the soldiers' need to believe in the justice of the war in which they are fighting and in the way the war is being conducted, as well as the soldiers' faith in the uncompromising commitment of those who have sent them to war: the military and the state as a whole.

Israeli society's prevailing belief that the conflict with the Palestinians has reached an impasse demands that we face up to the new risk factors for CSR and combat PTSD inasmuch as that belief presupposes a need to reinforce the resilience of soldiers. The current atmosphere in Israel makes it very hard to engage in such a self-accounting. The various approaches to the issue cut across ideological lines and cannot be identified with this or that end of the political spectrum. Regarding, for example, the POW-MIA issue, a hawkish attitude toward fighting the Palestinians often coexists with the view that the state should limit its commitment to evacuating soldiers stranded behind enemy lines, given the perception that such evacuations exact a heavy national "price." In other words, an expectation that supporters of intensified military activity would demonstrate a stronger commitment to soldiers left in the field is not borne out by the current reality. On the contrary, militants frequently oppose what they perceive as capitulating to the enemy in order to bring POWs and MIAs home. This attitude is based both on a resurgence of old myths that emphasize the individual's complete self-sacrifice on behalf of the collective and on a mistaken assumption that soldiers, by laying their lives on the line, are authorizing state and society to refrain from paying too high a "price" for their return home. This assumption implies that some of the Israeli public identifies the expectation of the state's outright commitment to the soldier with weakness, which may help explain the difficulty in coming to terms with the fact that the absence of such commitment constitutes a risk factor for CSR and combat PTSD.

Moral injury (transparent trauma) is another issue that arouses opposition on both ends of the political spectrum. The more militant Israelis generally see it as defamation of the IDF, since it hints at inappropriate conduct on the army's part. A vociferous number of far-left Israelis view the claims of moral injury as verbal whitewashing replacing concrete resistance activity, in the form of refusal to take part in the occupation. These Israelis oppose recognizing the trauma of the soldier who inflicts harm on others, because they see such recognition as an evasion of moral responsibility. In their view, the soldier should have disobeyed the order that led to his trauma, or even refused to serve in the territories. Soldiers who do not refuse are, according to them, partners in the Occupation apparatus who use their trauma to absolve themselves of blame after the fact.

The rare convergence of critics and supporters of war, from the left and the right, on the issue of moral injury hampers meaningful discussion, not only of moral conflict as a risk factor for CSR and combat PTSD, but also of the very fact that military activity is being conducted within a civilian population. Both political factions leave soldiers to cope in isolation with policies that they have no hand in shaping and whose implementation they have the moral burden of bearing. This contradictory consensus regarding the dismissal of transparent trauma obscures the moral responsibility of Israeli society as a whole for that which is done in its name.

Notes

1. On the relationship between army and society in Israel see Peri (2007); Sheffer (2008).
2. The army-settler clashes have been covered extensively by the Israeli press. One article that effectively conveys the dilemmas with which the IDF is faced in such situations, and the quandary in which the army finds itself, is Caspit (2005).

3. A bitter and long-standing dispute has subsisted between the bereaved families and the Ministry of Defense regarding rights to the body of the fallen soldier and to the information pertaining to him, in life and death, as well as rights to his grave. Currently, the information belongs to the family (except where special security needs come into play), the corpse belongs to the family (in the sense of having the right to take leave of it under any conditions), and the place of interment belongs jointly to the state and to the family, with rights divided between the tombstone and the grave itself. As explained to the author by Professor Avraham (Rami) Friedman, who performed reserve duty for many years with the IDF's Casualties Department, 3 September 2009 (henceforth Friedman interview, 2009).
4. www.izkor.gov.il/HalalKorot.aspx?id=515713, retrieved 12 June 2010. [Hebrew]
5. The sentence is quoted in the explanatory material accompanying Yotam Reuveny's "Ballad of Yusuf Madhat," which includes a passage from a letter disseminated to IDF soldiers by Chief Education Office Elazar Stern and Combat Doctrine Division head Gershon Hacohen.
6. Reservists founded a movement called *Ichpat* [We care] and organized demonstrations against the IDF high command, the prime minister, and the minister of defense. See *Ynet*, 8 July 2002, www.ynet.co.il/articles/1,7340,L-1985474,00.html, retrieved 6 December 2009. [Hebrew]
7. For an extensive discussion of Israel's efforts to bring home POWs and MIAs, see Bergman (2009).
8. For a detailed discussion of the failures of the Second Lebanon War and the points of controversy that it raised, see "The Commission of Inquiry into the Events of Military Engagement in Lebanon, 2006." The commission was headed by Judge Eliyahu Winograd, and its members were Professor Yehezkel Dror, Professor Ruth Gabizon, General (Res.) Chaim Nadel, and General (Res.) Menachem Enan. The commission's appointment document and the reports that it produced may be viewed online at www.vaadatwino.co.il/reports.html. Retrieved 12 June 2010 (henceforth Winograd Commission Report). [Hebrew]
9. Winograd Commission Report, Final Report, January 2008, p. 355, comment 12.
10. Author's correspondence with Miri Shalit, director of the Dan Region of RDMD, July 2011.
11. Shalit interview, 2008.
12. For an in-depth discussion of Israel's efforts to bring POWs and MIAs home, see Bergman (2009).
13. On the efforts to bring about Arad's release, see ibid.
14. The Shamgar Committee, chaired by Meir Shamgar, former president of the Supreme Court, was formed in 2009, after public criticism and debate over POW exchanges carried out by Israel in the past. Among them was the deal in 2004, in which the bodies of Adi Avitan, Omar Souad, and Benny Avraham together with the (alive) citizen Elhanan Tannenbaum were returned to Israel for 436 Palestinian and Lebanese terrorists, including Mustafa Dirani and Sheikh Abdul Karim Obeid. Another deal was signed in 2008 in which bodies of reservists Eldad Regev and Ehud Goldwasser were returned for 197 bodies of Hezbollah fighters, and 5 Palestinian and Lebanese prisoners, one of whom was the infamous Samir Kuntar, a terrorist who, in 1979, entered Israeli northern town of Naharia through the sea, abducted four Israeli citizens from their homes, and murdered them. Among them was a four-year-old girl, Einat Haran, whose head he smashed with a rock after shooting her father in front of her. The need to set clear rules became more acute during the months preceding the Gilad Shalit deal, and it was determined that the recommendations of the committee would serve as the guidelines in the case of future negotiations, but not in the case of Shalit. The committee report has been kept confidential.
15. All of Ehud Barak's quoted statements regarding Gilad Shalit are from a news report on Barak's remarks during an encounter with high school students in southern Israel

on 19 August 2009: "Barak: Don't Preach to Me about Shalit's Release," NRG *Maariv*, News Edition: Political-Diplomatic, 2 September, retrieved 13 September 2009 from www.nrg.co.il/online/1/ART1/937/549.html.

16. Author's interview with attorney Uri Slonim, 11 February 2009. Adv. Slonim served as advisor to the minister of defense on POW-MIA issues during the period 1989–2000, and worked strenuously to bring about the return of Ron Arad. He was also involved in the efforts to secure Gilad Shalit's release. I thank him for his willingness to take part in the interview, which expanded my knowledge and understanding of the POW-MIA issue.

References

Bar-Tal, D. 2007, *Living with the Conflict: Socio-Psychological Analysis of Jewish Society in Israel*, Carmel, Jerusalem.

Bergman, R. 2009, *By Any Means Necessary: Israel's Covert War for Its POWs and MIAs*, Kinneret Zmora-Bitan Dvir, Or Yehuda. (Hebrew)

Caspit, B. 2005, 'On the Brink of the Abyss', NRG *Maariv*, 8 July.

IDF Manpower Directorate 2000. 'Yoseph's Tomb – Values and Discretion', 6 December. Available from www.aka.idf.il/chinuch/klali/default.asp?catId=42844&docId=48305 [6 December 2009]. (Hebrew)

Keynan, I. 2008, 'The Price of Not Releasing the Captured Soldier', *Ynet*, 24 June.

Lyotard, J.-F. 1979, *The Postmodern Condition*, Manchester University Press, Manchester.

May Every Mother Know [*Teda Kol Em*] 2007, documentary film.

Morris, B. 1989, *The Birth of the Palestinian Refugee Problem, 1947–1949*, Cambridge University Press, Cambridge.

Peri, Y. 2007, 'Cosmetic or Real Changes? Media-Defense Relations at the Turn of the 21st Century', *Media Frameworks*, vol. 1, pp. 153–168. (Hebrew)

Reuveny, Y. n.d., 'Ballad of Yusuf Madhat'. Available from www.nymrod.info/1112.htm [6 December 2009]. (Hebrew)

Rosenthal, R. 2001, *Is Bereavement Dead?*, Keter, Jerusalem. (Hebrew)

Sheffer, G. 2008, 'Army-Society Relations in Israel', *Politika: the Israeli Journal of Political Science and International Relations*, vol. 1, pp. 183–196. (Hebrew)

Yonah, Y. 2005, *In Virtue of Difference: the Multicultural Project in Israel*, Van Leer Institute and Hakibbutz Hameuchad, Jerusalem. (Hebrew)

Zakai, S. 2009, interview, *Channel 2 News*, 6 November.

Part II

The Israeli Home Front

Between Heroism and Victimhood*

**A note on the terminology used in this part of the book:*

The term "victims of hostile acts" appeared in reference to civilians for the first time in the Compensation for Victims of Hostile Acts Law, drafted in September 1969 and enacted in 1970. The term "hostilities-related injury" may refer to an injury incurred from a hostile act perpetrated by enemy forces, an inadvertent injury that occurred in the context of a hostile act, or an injury from a violent act aimed at harming a person because of the victim's ethnic-religious background, in connection with the Israeli-Arab conflict. The precise definition of the term used in the law is available on the National Insurance Institute (NII) website: www.btl.gov.il/English%20Homepage/Benefits/Benefits%20for%20Victims%20of%20Hostilities/Pages/default.aspx#anchorSpan_517a9b2b2e1e4b23a93f7f2a6b853a6b.

The difference between situations defined as "war" and those defined as "hostile acts" is of great significance for the types of benefits provided by the state, but is not relevant to our present discussion. I will therefore employ the term "victims of hostile acts" or "victims of hostilities" to refer to all civilians injured in security incidents arising from the Israeli-Palestinian conflict, with no distinction between war situations and other hostile incidents that do not fall into the category of war. The Hebrew term employed by Israel's NII in reference to civilians suffering from traumatic injury or acute stress is "anxiety casualties." I will refer to the implications of this phrasing later in this part. The English term the NII uses is "emotional trauma casualties" (www.btl.gov.il/English%20Homepage/Publications/AnnualSurvey/2007/Documents/chap-4–08-ENG.pdf, box 14). This term encompasses both those afflicted with acute stress reaction and those suffering from PTSD; the difference between the two is explained in the introduction to this volume. For brevity's sake, I will generally employ the terms "acute stress," "ACR," "trauma," and "PTSD" as general terms to describe all manifestations of traumatic and post-traumatic disorders among civilians.

7 Lower in Rank

Israeli Citizens in War and Terror

Israeli Hierarchy of Heroism

Overshadowed by constant threats to national security, Israeli civilian life has always been fraught with tension. Every few years these threats flare into war—large or small—and even the intervening periods of relative peace are punctuated by hostile acts, mostly against civilians. Since the founding of the state, over 3,000 incidents, excluding wars, have been recognized in Israel as hostile acts, resulting in more than 20,000 civilian casualties and 2,000 civilian deaths.[1] It is unknown precisely how many among these casualties suffered from acute stress reactions (ASR) and PTSD because no government data were collected before 2006, with the exception of the Gulf War, during which over 500 acute stress civilian casualties were reported. In the Second Lebanon War of 2006, the National Insurance Institute (NII) reported 1,870 civilians suffering from acute stress with no physical injury, 37% of the total number of civilians wounded in the war (Baer 2007, Table 16, p. 23).[2] While most will recover, 1 in 12 (8.5%) are likely to develop PTSD (Somer & Bleich 2005).

Since the first waves of Zionist immigration in the late 1800s, a social norm emerged among Israelis, dictating that civilians carry on with their daily lives wherever they are and whatever the conditions, and display fortitude and bravery in the face of external threats. At the same time, the expectation that civilians act like "soldiers without uniforms"—a very common phrase in Israel—stood in stark contrast to the lack of government and public acknowledgment of their sacrifice in the event of their injury or death. This contradiction corresponds to Israel's traditional "scale of bereavement and heroism," on which civilian victims of war and hostile acts occupy secondary status,[3] and which performs significant formal and informal social functions in Israeli society. Informally, society offers victims differential levels of social support, a sense of obligation to care for survivors and bereaved families, and public appreciation of their sacrifice. These meaningful factors in coping with the personal tragedy are allotted differently, according to whether the public perceives the context of the casualty as the battlefield or the civilian home front. The formal implications of the heroism scale are related to official commemoration of those killed, with a clear distinction between soldiers and civilians, and to state-established criteria that differentiate between the rights and benefits of the soldiers and those of civilians injured and their families.[4] Chapter 11 shows that most Western countries distinguish between civilian and military casualties. In Israel, however, in the last two decades, this distinction has become the subject of a bitter debate over recognition of civilian suffering caused by war or terrorist attacks.

Unlike most Western and European countries whose soldiers fight in different places around the world, but whose civilians have not been exposed to wars since World War II, targeting Israeli citizens has become an integral element in the enemy's objectives, especially since the 1990s.

During the first 50 years of Israeli statehood, the traditional hierarchy of heroism and the inferior position of civilians on this scale were supported by a strong public consensus, which was based on the centrality of the heroism ethos in Israel's life. However, once warfare spread to the home front, especially with the deadly terrorist attacks of the late 1990s and the Al-Aqsa Intifada, the distinction between soldiers at the dangerous front and civilians at the relatively secure home front began to weaken. Increasingly, the hierarchy of heroism has become the focus of a bitter and painful dispute between the bereaved families of fallen soldiers, who seek to preserve soldiers' higher status on this hierarchy, and the families of civilians killed in hostile acts, who firmly believe that the losses suffered by both groups should be afforded equal respect, honor, and standing.

Gradually, as a result of concurrent paths, a change began in the status of victims of hostile acts, as a group. The official path comprises increasing formal state recognition of its responsibility for injured citizens and organizational efforts by the injured themselves, through groups like the Terror Victims Association, while the unofficial path encompasses efforts to secure the status of civilians within Israel's hierarchy of heroism and maintains a vigorous public debate around this issue. Specifically, victims of hostile acts and their families have sought to escape their secondary status in the Israeli heroism discourse, demanding to view sacrifice by civilians as a conscious act, one embodying a dedication and willingness to risk one's life comparable to that of a soldier.

Government and public recognition of individual war trauma among civilians emerged in line with similar changes in perception within the army. This recognition came about through the advancement of knowledge, both locally and globally, of the intensity and scope of psychological trauma caused by war, natural disaster, and terrorist attacks. Despite similar symptomologies, combat PTSD and civilian trauma triggered profoundly different attitudes in Israeli society. The fact that civilian psychological trauma began to attract public attention precisely at a time when the home front was under frequent attack resulted in increasingly polarized attitudes toward this form of injury. Together with growing compassion for the sufferers of psychological trauma of war, a rhetoric of resilience gained currency in Israel. Politicians and opinion makers increasingly called for individual resolve and displays of fortitude, behavior construed as essential to national security and to patriotism. Thus, on one hand, the large number of civilians killed and injured, including the emotionally traumatized, supported the idea of equivalence between the scope of hurt and sacrifice of civilians and soldiers on Israel's hierarchy of heroism. On the other hand, the fact that so many of the wounded civilians are mentally injured, in numbers exceeding the physically injured, reinforced their inferior position on the scale. The stress wound is still considered inferior, and less than a "genuine" injury.

If we are to understand how attitudes toward acute stress of civilians have evolved in Israel, we first need to understand state and social attitudes toward civilian war casualties in general. The present part of the book opens with an analysis of this issue, about which very little has yet been written. It addresses the place occupied by civilians on the Israeli hierarchy of heroism and their struggle to assert their equivalence to soldiers, and then offers a comprehensive review of how the changing character of the Israeli-Palestinian conflict and the spread of warfare to the home front have made the issue of acute stress casualties a central topic of public debate. Special attention is given to the Gulf War and the Al-Aqsa Intifada, each of which had a major impact on attitudes toward civilian war trauma and PTSD and on the dialectical interaction between the trauma discourse and the discourse of national resilience. This part of the book concludes with a discussion of trauma in Arab society (Chapter 12), a sector of the population that usually remains at the margins of Jewish-Israeli public awareness.

Victims and Heroes: A Vise of Contradictions—Is the Entire Country a War Front, the Entire Nation an Army?

During the early months of Israel's War of Independence, war front and home front merged, and civilian life was profoundly affected by the war. The battlefield was everywhere, in rural areas and in major cities. Even when the war front began to recede from main residential areas, six months into the fighting, Jerusalem and many rural localities remained in the line of fire (Bar-On & Hazan 2010). This situation gave rise to the expression, "the entire country is a war front, the entire nation an army," a general zeitgeist that faded from Israeli memory in later years, once the Israel Defense Forces (IDF) succeeded in establishing a military doctrine that maintained that fighting should take place across the border.

Following the War of Independence, the attitude of Israeli society toward civilian casualties was shaped by two major factors: a clear distinction between battlefield and civilian population, and different rank in the scale of heroism attributed to injured soldiers and civilians. In Israel's first two decades, this cultural attitude was manifested in the extent of state assistance to those afflicted by war: different benefits and caring resources granted to injured soldiers and civilians.

For 42 years—from the end of the War of Independence (July 1949) to the first Gulf War (1991)—a clear distinction between war front and home front was successfully maintained, and civilian society's role was limited to providing support and morale, admittedly vital resources for effective fighting. Civilians went on with their daily lives; they expressed faith in, and support for, the IDF; and they maintained a willingness to send their loved ones to war despite fears for their safety.[5] The occasional infiltrations and security breaches into towns and cities did not fracture the relative sense of security that civilians experienced, further underscoring their reliance on the army. For this reason, the secondary status of civilians on the heroism scale remained unquestioned for many years. Heroism, a concept that played a central role in the national ethos, was contingent upon a sense of mission and an element of intention to risk one's life in defense of the country. According to the criterion of intent, soldiers consciously endanger their lives to ensure the nation's survival and the security of life on the home front, and therefore, when they sacrifice their lives or are injured, they occupy the highest rung on the ladder of heroism, higher than that accorded to civilians. While civilians may be targeted purely on account of being Israeli, such injuries take place within the context of their daily life. A civilian's presence at the scene of an attack, whether on a bus, in a café, or on the way to work, is coincidental. Missing from the civilian experience of injury is the central motif of intent—a conscious self-sacrifice for the good of the nation, which alone can entitle one to the esteem and gratitude of the collective and the state.

In accordance with the inferior status of nonuniformed victims of war on the nation's heroism scale, the government assumed limited responsibility for the welfare of injured civilians, establishing asymmetry between an individual's duty to the collective and the collective's responsibility toward the individual. Such a short time after the Holocaust, Israelis' attitude towards the Jewish state was of unquestioning reverence, as the ultimate representative of the collective. The state of Israel was considered to be the only shield against anti-Semitism and the only thing that could ensure a free national existence, which contained within it individual liberty. After 2,000 years of persecution, Israelis, many of them refugees, vested in the independent Jewish State a formidable, almost sacred, significance. These feelings reflect Erikson's (1995) description of the euphoria felt by trauma survivors when they realize that their community survived after all. In such cases, the commitment to the continuity of the community is so strong that it overshadows the individual's needs and rights. In newly born Israel, this paradigm overemphasized the individual's duties as the only way to guarantee the nation's continued safety and independence, and fueled social norms of personal fortitude, a "stiff upper lip," and refusal to reveal weakness or pain, lest the enemy rejoice and attack again, thinking it can win. Fortitude was the duty of all members of society: civilians, soldiers, and bereaved families, who were expected to bear their pain in silence, with restraint and pride, and to reconcile themselves to the somewhat consolatory idea that their children had sacrificed their young lives "on the altar of [national] redemption."[6] At the same time, these norms also constrained governmental responsibility for injured civilians.

The emergency regulations of the 1949 Repair of War Damage and Houses Ordinance vested the Ministry of War Casualties with the responsibility of dealing with physically injured civilians, damaged property, evacuees, and the provision of services to war-wounded civilians. Although the operations of the Ministry of War Casualties during the War of Independence had been guided by the principle that "anyone injured in war is entitled to compensation and assistance,"[7] entitlement was not based on the state's universal obligation to its injured citizens. With the state's then-precarious finances, and in accordance with the prevailing philosophy of the time, citizens were expected to seek aid or compensation from the government only as a last resort. "The Ministry is unable to adequately compensate large property owners," noted the daily newspaper *HaTzofe*, and therefore "public companies and large property owners should defer their claims until a later time . . . The Ministry offers assistance to people who are homeless and destitute."[8] As a result, governmental assistance was something exceptional, granted only in specific instances of great need, "as a gesture of charity, at the discretion of the Minister."[9]

This approach to compensation as charity rather than obligation is also reflected in the decision, taken at the time of the Ministry's dissolution in 1951, to transfer matters pertaining to civilian war casualties to the Ministry of Welfare. The transfer was stipulated in the War Damage Compensation Tax Law of 1951 and brought about no real change in the way aid was provided to injured civilians. The law conferred no universal right to benefits, and the discretionary power to grant assistance, and to specify its amount, was left to the directors of the local welfare departments (Yanay 1995). This measure all but equated victims of hostile acts with welfare recipients, a categorization reinforced by the requirement imposed on wounded civilians and bereaved families to prove their financial need. In other words, the state saw civilian injury from a hostile act as personal tragedy rather than an event of national significance for which the state should take responsibility. Moreover, the wounded civilian, classified as a welfare recipient, was thus branded a passive victim of fate—sometimes even as a parasite, and certainly not as a hero entitled to the state's gratitude. This attitude, which highlighted the distinction between military and civilian victims of hostile acts, reinforced the latter's inferior status on the heroism scale.

Left to the discretion of regional directors, and because eligibility for aid was based on financial need rather than clear and uniform tests related to the injury itself, bereaved or injured civilians often qualified for very different levels of assistance, despite having lost loved ones in incidents of a similar nature or suffering similar types or degrees of disability. This lack of uniformity persisted not only between welfare offices in different localities but also sometimes within the same office (ibid.). Although the aid provided to victims of hostile acts was usually more substantial than that accorded to other welfare recipients, in the eyes of the state they were no different.

"We Are a Generation That Inhabits the Land": Frontier Towns[10] as War Front or Home Front

Despite the clear distinction between soldiers and civilians, one group of civilians did win the status of quasi-soldiers in the eyes of the public and on the ladder of heroism. These were the residents of the frontiers, where skirmishes in the 1950s escalated in intensity as the decade wore on. Forty-five Israelis were killed and murdered and dozens of others injured in repeated infiltrations by Fedayeen[11] from the neighboring countries. Israel responded with retaliatory strikes that grew ever harsher, to the point of sparking domestic debate over their intensity and scope (Zertal 2002).[12]

On April 29, 1956, a young man named Ro'i Rutenberg was killed on the Israeli side of the Gaza Strip border. Ro'i was shot in an ambush while riding his horse in the fields of kibbutz Nahal Oz, where he had gone to live in the framework of a *garin* (literally, *seed*), a quasi-military group that spent a part of its military service living in and establishing frontier towns and villages on Israel's borders. Over time, these *garins*, whose location was dictated by national security conditions, developed into civilian towns and villages where many *garin* members settled permanently after they completed their military service. Ro'i's body was desecrated by the attackers and returned only after UN mediation. Moshe Dayan, Israel's acclaimed general, who at that time was in charge of Southern Israel, had visited Kibbutz Nahal Oz a short time before the violent incident and had been deeply impressed by the Nahal pioneers. Ro'i's death shocked Dayan particularly, as he recalled from his visit the young man "with light in his heart," almost a child, who had come from Tel Aviv to build his home on Israel's southern border. The eulogy that he delivered for Ro'i became an oft-quoted text, which seemed to express the sentiments of the entire nation. It reflects beliefs that had been prevalent in Israel from the time of its founding and the vise of contradictions that ensnares civilians injured in war and hostile acts.[13]

The story of Ro'i Rutenberg's life and death tragically illustrates the ambiguity of the frontier areas as a military and civil category, and the ambiguous attitude toward civilians injured in security incidents during the 1950s and 1960s. Was Ro'i a soldier or a civilian? Dayan's eulogy does not at first describe him as a soldier prepared to meet the enemy, but rather as a civilian, even a boy, who encountered murderers as he went out to breathe the fresh air of the fields: "The quiet of the spring morning dazzled him and he did not see those waiting in ambush for him at the edge of the furrow." However, Dayan proceeded to ascribe to Rutenberg qualities of an explicitly soldierly nature, noting that he had gone to the border out of a conscious sense of mission, assuming his role of defender of civilians: he went to "the gates of Gaza to be a wall for us." Dayan saw the conflation of Ro'i's civilian and military identities as a natural one, dictated by the circumstances: "We are a generation that inhabits the land, and without the steel helmet and the cannon's maw, we will not be able to plant a tree and build a home." For those belonging to this generation, Dayan continued, war was destiny, something that had to be reconciled as "our life's choice." One needed to be "prepared and armed, strong and determined, lest the sword be stricken from our fist and our lives cut down" (Dayan, 1976, p. 190).

This was by no means an unusual way of looking at things. The idea that the civilian border towns and villages served to defend the state, that their inhabitants fulfilled the mission of both reclaiming the land and defending the country, was consistent with the time-honored Israeli ethos of "redeeming" or regaining control of the land through agricultural work. This ethos had existed since the earliest period of Zionist inhabitation in Eretz Yisrael[14] and would remain valid for many years after the death of Ro'i Rutenberg. As evidenced in an impassioned statement by Knesset member Ada Sereni during a debate on the status of the frontier residents 13 years later, inhabiting the land and defending it were fully enmeshed with the nation's existential struggle. Comparing those who settled the border areas to soldiers, Sireni stated, "That farmer who goes out to pick the cotton in an area beyond the IDF patrol road, that moshav (an agricultural community very common in Israel) resident who goes out to milk the cows at night, that child who sleeps night after night in the shelter—they are full-fledged soldiers."[15]

In 1956, these beliefs gained official endorsement for the first time with the enactment of the Benefits for Border Casualties Law, which established "border communities" as a special category eligible to certain privileges, benefits, and help from the government. According to this law, victims of hostile acts or their survivors residing or active in these border localities were eligible for compensation.[16] (While the settlements beyond the Green Line, in the territories occupied in the Six-Day War, claimed the same legitimacy as other settlements, they have not gained the same level of public support.)

The 1956 law partially resolved the contradiction inherent in the long-standing tradition that viewed border inhabitants, farmers, and pioneers as soldiers in the fullest sense of the term yet failed to grant them the same rights as soldiers.[17] It transferred the responsibility for border casualties from the Welfare Ministry to the NII, and cancelled the income test and the burden-of-proof requirement that had applied earlier to injured civilians, who had to demonstrate that their injuries had indeed been caused by hostile acts (Yanay 1995).[18] However, the law did not elevate the rights of civilian border casualties to the level of wounded armed forces personnel; civilian border casualties would be eligible only for the degree of practical assistance available to victims of work-related injuries. The law's many deficiencies notwithstanding, it constituted a major Israeli socio-legal milestone: from that point on, the state openly acknowledged its responsibility toward civilians injured in security incidents, though not in all parts of the country.[19] This law, which, for the first time, distinguished the border-casualty population from welfare recipients and other individuals with disabilities, marked official recognition of their contribution to the state, consequently elevating them to a higher rung on the bereavement and heroism ladder. However, differentiation of border casualties from other civilian casualties, whose status remained on par with welfare recipients, had the unfortunate consequence of creating more rather than fewer categories of heroism and entitlement.

Neither the Benefits for Border Casualties Law of 1956 nor the law enacted in the following decade, expressing the state's full responsibility for the material well-being of victims of hostile acts, made mention of civilians suffering war-related emotional trauma. During the 1950s, 1960s, and 1970s, the incidence of war trauma, whether of civilians or soldiers, was consistently suppressed or denied, and psychological injuries caused by war-related events were not even a subject of discussion.

The Heroism Scale during the Transition from Charity to Rights

It took an additional 14 years before the Compensation for Victims of Hostile Acts Law of 1970 created parity between the rights and social benefits accorded to victims of hostile acts and their families and those of wounded armed forces personnel. The change took place against the growing frequency of hostile acts and rising numbers of victims after the Six-Day War, as well as the spread of such acts to central Israel and even to Israeli facilities abroad, including airlines.[20] The law invalidated distinctions based on the geographic site of the injury—border communities or elsewhere—and expanded the definition of "hostile acts" in a way that would make it easier for the injured to substantiate their claims (Yanay 1995).[21] Ultimately, the new law led to the institutionalization of eligibility for aid from the state as a universal right, in cases of injury at enemy hands—regardless of whether the injured party was a uniformed member of the armed forces and regardless of his or her place of residence.[22] The law's greatest achievement, however, was its symbolic significance: official and public recognition that a civilian injury caused by hostile acts is not a random, personal tragedy but rather a part of the cost of war borne by the nation as a whole.

Surprising as it may appear, the equalization of the benefits received by civilian victims of hostile acts and soldiers did not fundamentally alter the inferior societal ranking of civilians on the Israeli scale of heroism. This was reflected, for example, in the conflict between the NII—the entity responsible for implementing the law—and the Ministry of Defense, each deflecting financial responsibility for the victims onto the other through administrative and theoretical arguments.[23] Arguing on administrative considerations, the NII insisted that, since the relevant information and the authority to grant and update rights and benefits remained in the Defense Ministry's hands, the Ministry should take responsibility for assisting civilian victims of hostile acts, now that their rights had been equalized. The Defense Ministry, in turn, offered administrative and budgetary counterarguments. However, both entities also raised theoretical arguments that clearly reflected conflicting ideological views regarding civilians' ranking on the heroism scale. The NII claimed that victims of hostile acts were not content with equal financial rights, but rather sought the full public recognition of their status that could be conferred only through affiliation with the Defense Ministry. The Ministry argued to preserve the universal practice of distinguishing between soldier and civilian, through various means, including the army's responsibility for uniformed casualties alone (ibid.). Ultimately, the Defense Ministry's position prevailed, and to this day the NII handles civilian victims of hostile acts. Israel's legislators thereby affirmed that the state views its soldiers as the bearers of a unique national mission and extols their willingness to pursue this mission and consciously endanger their lives for the sake of the nation. The reasons for the persistent distinction between soldiers' and civilians' rank on the ladder of heroism may be the result of the popular admiration for the army and its central role in war-stricken Israel, especially after the victory of the 1967 Six-Day War. The 1973 Yom Kippur War further reaffirmed the well-defined division of labor between the civilian population and the army, and the critical role that soldiers' acts of heroism played in saving the country from a catastrophe.

A clear distinction between war front and home front still prevailed when the First Lebanon War broke out (1982), as did the conventional attribution to soldiers of conscious intent and sense of mission while risking their lives to ensure the safety of civilians. The very name chosen for the first Lebanon war, "Operation Peace for the Galilee," symbolized this consensus, which persisted in Israel despite bitter debates over the war's goals, justification, and outcomes. The Israeli government maintained that the army had been sent into Lebanon so that the children and parents of the Galilee could live in peace and security. In the view of Prime Minister Menachem Begin, the IDF had thereby fulfilled not only the mission that every army of every democratic state is expected to fulfill but also the unique mission entrusted to the IDF—serving as a buffer between the State of Israel and the age-old Jewish fate of persecution and powerlessness. "The fate of a million and a half Jewish children differed from that of all children around the world, in all generations," said Begin before the Israeli parliament (Knesset). "No longer. We will defend our children."[24] Begin linked the current situation to the Jewish people's collective memory, evoking feelings of colossal threat and the Holocaust. "You know what I have done[25] and what we all have done in order to prevent war and bereavement," he said to the Cabinet of Israel on the eve of the IDF's entry into Lebanon, "but it is our fate that in Eretz Yisrael there is no choice but to fight with total devotion. Believe me, the alternative is Treblinka, and we have decided that there will never be another Treblinka."[26]

Begin's words encapsulate widely held Israeli beliefs about the existential threat to which Jews are exposed on account of their nationality—and the unassailable role of the State of Israel and the IDF in repelling this threat. These beliefs in an existential threat are not mitigated by the sense of relative security enjoyed by civilians on the home front. On the contrary, their feeling of security is based on faith in the existence of a well-defined military apparatus that enables civilians to lead normal lives. These attitudes reinforce the appreciation, bordering at times on adulation, accorded to soldiers for their sacrifice—in contrast to the milder empathy elicited by civilian suffering, which is perceived as lower in value. Those who supported the First Lebanon War saw in it an affirmation of the need for a hierarchy of heroism, an incentive to soldiers to bear their dangerous burden of defending the home front and keeping the war front far away from civilians. Those who opposed the war did not reject the ethos of steadfastly defending the civilian population; they merely saw no real need for such defense at that particular time. From whatever perspective one views it, the First Lebanon War demonstrated more effectively than ever the sharp distinction between war front and home front and the army's role as defender: while soldiers were still being killed in Lebanon, with many others returning battle-shocked and emotionally and physically scarred, life within Israel's borders bore no traces of war.

Although it caused the death of 50 Jewish citizens, the First Intifada (1987–1993) in the West Bank, which took place while the army was still in Lebanon, did not shake the sense of relative security that prevailed on the Israeli home front.

This may have happened because most of the casualties were settlers in the occupied territories; the Intifada was not experienced as a threat to mainstream life in Israel (within the Green Line).[27]

Still, the public expressed considerable concern over this new type of war against terrorism. Public debates were sparked specifically by what the public perceived as the emotional toll and moral dilemmas experienced by soldiers engaged in a new form of combat, facing Palestinian civilians, including children and adolescents. Even though the military leadership rejected these concerns and attempted to downplay them and remove them from the public agenda, the public remained more concerned with the fate of the young soldiers than with the fate of settlers who were targets of Intifada attacks: the time was not ripe for challenging the status of civilians in the long-established heroism scale. Greater concern with civilian casualties would emerge only a decade later, when public opinion could no longer ignore the conflict's ever-deepening penetration into civilian population centers around the country, and the resulting incidence of acute stress in the civilian population.

Notes

1. According to the National Insurance Institute's "Annual Report for 2012" (2013), there have been 20,961 civilian casualties in hostile acts since 1948, including 1,840 dead. These figures do not include the most recent war against Hamas in Gaza in July–August 2014, which is taking place at the time of writing.
2. Maintaining statistics on emotional trauma casualties is a difficult matter. Many recover in time, on their own or with the aid of independently organized psychotherapy, while those who develop PTSD subsequent to their acute stress injury, or who experience delayed-onset PTSD, are not always known to or recognized by the authorities. Again, these figures do not include the latest war against Hamas in Gaza in July–August 2014. After approximately one month of fighting, the Israeli Ministry of Health announced that more than 600 Israeli civilians were suffering from acute stress injury.
3. See www.vaadatgoren.gov.il. See also Schwartz et al. (2005).
4. In recent years, the Ministry of Defense has called attention to yet another hierarchy, one within the military, ranking fallen and wounded IDF soldiers according to how the fatality or injury occurred. Relevant to this issue is the public committee appointed by the Israeli government in 2009, under the leadership of Judge Uri Goren, the Goren Committee. The Committee was asked to examine the eligibility criteria for assistance from the Disabled Rehabilitation Division and the Department of Families and Remembrance in order to "enhance efficiency and ensure savings within the rehabilitation system." The Committee was instructed to strive for a "distinction between those injured during the course of their service due to activity of an operational nature and other casualties." Letter of nomination, signed by the prime minister and the minister of defense, 18 November 2009. Retrieved from http://www.vaadatgoren.gov.il/tabid/59/Default.aspx.
5. On the anxiety of having sent a son off to war, see Grossman (2008).
6. From a poem by Eleazar Kallir, father of a son who fell in the War of Independence. The poem appeared in the *Davar HaShavua*, a weekly supplement to *Davar*, 9 May 1951 (quoted in Azaryahu 1995, p. 111). (Published between 1925 [under the British Mandate] and May 1996, *Davar* represented the ideas and concepts of the labor party and was one the influential daily newspapers in Israel.) See also a statement by Ephraim E. Urbach, whose soldier son fell in the Six-Day War, at a conference held by the Public Council for Soldiers' Commemoration in 1975, on bereaved families' feeling that their

sorrow overshadowed the joy of victory in war. Professor Urbach's statement conveys families' sense of being implicitly expected to downplay their grief (Shamir 1976, p. 14). On changing approaches to bereavement in Israel, see Rosenthal (2001).

7. *HaTzofe* 1948, 5 September. *Hatzofe* was a daily Israeli newspaper, which stopped appearing on 2007. It declared its point of view as Zionist, nationalist, and religious.
8. Ibid.
9. Ibid.
10. In the years prior to 1967 the word "settlements" was used to represent small rural communities within the recognized boundaries of Israel, which were finalized in the 1949 Cease Fire Talks and are known today as the "Green Line border." These are completely different from the current use of the term "the settlements" to refer to Jewish localities in the occupied territories, beyond the Green Line. I chose the word "towns" in order to prevent confusion.
11. Militants or guerrillas of a nationalist orientation from among the Palestinian people, who made efforts to infiltrate Israeli territory to strike mostly civilian targets, in the aftermath of the 1949 Arab-Israeli cease-fire agreements.
12. Casualty data from Baer (2007, Table 2).
13. The complete text of the eulogy can be found in Dayan (1976, p. 190). The English version is available online at http://en.wikipedia.org/wiki/Nahal_Oz. Idith Zertal (2002) analyzes Dayan's eulogy for Rutenberg (ibid., p. 246) as one of two texts central to 1950s Israel, along with a state address by Ben-Gurion on 19 October 1953, following the slaughter carried out in the then-Jordanian village of Qibya by Unit 101 and a paratroop company under the command of Ariel Sharon.
14. Eretz Yisrael, the land of Israel, is the Hebrew name Jews used for the area of the British Mandate (1922–1948), until the birth of the State of Israel. The name comes from the Bible, the territory that God promised to Abraham. In other languages it is also called the Promised Land, or the Holy Land and the Land of Milk and Honey.
15. Statement made during a discussion of the eligibility of civilian victims of hostile acts for benefits similar to those of servicemen; MK Sereni concludes by remarking that these civilians "are entitled to benefits like IDF soldiers" (quoted in Yanay 1995).
16. From the Dinim VeOd website, a legal database, retrieved on 19 March 2009 from www.dinimveod.co.il [Hebrew].
17. The settler heroism myth did not apply to all border settlers. Settlements whose residents were new immigrants, for instance, did not usually fall into this category. This fact is crucial to any understanding of the development of Israel's social-class structure and its exclusionary processes. This, however, is tangential to the present topic.
18. Instead of the wounded civilian having to prove his case, the authority to grant eligibility for benefits was vested in an "authorizing officer" appointed by the minister of defense.
19. These deficiencies included: confusion between injuries caused by hostile acts and those sustained in the workplace; a failure to address the needs of nonborder-area civilians injured in hostile acts; a failure to address the needs of volunteers who had gone to border areas and been injured there; and more. The law also did not resolve such issues as how to determine the eligibility level of self-employed personnel and of homemakers who were neither salaried employees nor self-employed. See Yanay et al. (2005).
20. According to National Insurance Institute data, the period between the Six-Day War and the end of the 1970s witnessed 462 Israeli fatalities (including those killed in terrorist attacks outside Israel). Some of the attacks resulted in mass casualties, such as the Mahane Yehuda car bomb incident in Jerusalem in November 1968 (12 killed), the Avivim school bus massacre of May 1970 (12 killed, most of them children), and the Lod Airport massacre of May 1970 (25 killed). Retrieved 14 June 2009 from the National Insurance Institute memorial site: http://laad.btl.gov.il.
21. For complete definitions pertaining to hostile acts, see Baer (2007, p. 1). The law was changed and updated over the years. For an in-depth discussion of these changes see Yanay et al. (2005).

22. This equalization was specified only in the Knesset's second and third readings of the bill; it was not stipulated at the beginning of the legislative process.
23. Deliberations of the Knesset Labor Committee, 17 January 1973 and 4 February 1973, per Yanay (1995).
24. Ninety-fifth meeting of the tenth Knesset, Tuesday, 8 June 1982, statement of Prime Minister Menachem Begin.
25. Begin refers here to the peace treaty with Egypt in 1979.
26. Cabinet meeting just prior to the IDF's entry into Lebanon (quoted in Naor 1986).
27. The First Intifada ceased almost completely after the Gulf War, but officially ended only with the signing of the Oslo Accords on September 1993. During the First Intifada 93 Israelis were killed: 47 adult civilians, 3 minors, and 43 soldiers. In that same period 1,070 Palestinians were killed, 237 of them minors. Data from the B'Tselem website: www.btselem.org/hebrew/Statistics/First_Intifada_Tables.asp. Retrieved 14 June 2009 [Hebrew] [English version at: www.btselem.org/statistics/first_intifada_tables].

References

Azaryahu, M. 1995, *State Cults: Celebrating Independence and Commemorating the Fallen in Israel 1948–1956*, Ben-Gurion University of the Negev Press, Be'er-Sheva. (Hebrew)

Baer, S. 2007, *Recipients of Hostile Acts Benefits, 2006*, National Insurance Institute, Research and Planning Administration. Available from www.btl.gov.il/Publications/survey%5CPages/Seker212.aspx.

Bar-On, M., & Hazan, M. (eds.) 2010, *Citizens at War: Studies on Civilian Society during the Israeli War of Independence*, Yad Yitzhak Ben-Zvi, Tel Aviv University, and the Galili Center for Defense Studies, Tel Aviv. (Hebrew)

Dayan, M. 1976, *Story of My Life*, Idanim, Jerusalem. (Hebrew)

Erikson, K. 1995, 'Notes on Trauma and Community', in *Trauma: Explorations in Memory*, ed. C. Caruth, Johns Hopkins University Press, Baltimore, pp. 183–199.

Grossman, D. 2008, *To the End of the Land*, Hakibbutz Hameuhad, Hasifriya Hahadasha, Tel Aviv. (Hebrew)

Naor, A. 1986, *Cabinet at War: the Functioning of the Israeli Cabinet during the Lebanon War (1982)*, Yedioth Ahronoth, Tel Aviv. (Hebrew)

National Insurance Institute 2013, *Annual Report for 2012*. Available from www.btl.gov.il/Publications/Skira_shnatit/2012/Documents/eiva.pdf [30 October 2013]. (Hebrew)

Rosenthal, R. 2001, *Is Bereavement Dead?*, Keter, Jerusalem. (Hebrew)

Schwartz, O. N., Lichtenreit, R., & Rubin, S. 2005, 'Bereavement, Ranking and Exclusion in Israel'. Paper presented at the Sderot Conference for Society, Sderot.

Shamir, I. (ed.) 1976, *Commemoration and Its Meaning: Issues in the Commemoration of Fallen IDF Soldiers*, Ministry of Defense, Rehabilitation Division, Tel Aviv. (Hebrew)

Somer, E., & Bleich, A. 2005, 'Stress in a Population under Prolonged Terrorist Attack: Identification, Characterization and Treatment Challenges' in *Mental Health in Terror's Shadow: the Israeli Experience*, eds. E. Somer & A. Bleich, Ramot, Tel Aviv, pp. 9–26. (Hebrew)

Yanay, U. 1995, 'Assistance to Civilian Victims of Hostile Acts', *Social Security*, vol. 40, pp. 35–53. (Hebrew)

Yanay, U., Prior, R., & Baer, S. 2005, *Victims of Hostile Acts in Israel: Injuries, Needs, Legislation and the Delivery of Services and Assistance*, School of Social Work, Hebrew University, and the Research and Planning Authority, the National Insurance Institute, Jerusalem. (Hebrew)

Zertal, I. 2002, *Death and the Nation: History, Memory, Politics*, Dvir, Or Yehuda. (Hebrew)

8 The Changing Face of War and the Emergence of a Trauma Discourse

The First Gulf War: National Trauma or War-Induced Trauma?

> In January 1991, Israel found itself in a terrifyingly unfamiliar military situation. The population came under attack from Iraqi missiles, suspected of being loaded with unconventional warheads, which threatened widespread devastation and reawakened the nation's deep-seated fears of annihilation. At the request of an American-led coalition force, Israel refrained from retaliating. This decision created a situation unique in Israeli military history: the primary military threat targeted the country's home front, while Israel's soldiers sat idly in their bases, concerned for their loved ones at home. Thus, this war awakened repressed fears of an impending existential threat to the country. As Lazarus (1986) showed, this offered a stark contrast with Israel's customary active response in the face of military threats—a traditionally essential component in Israelis' sense of security.[1]

The types of casualties of the Gulf War were also unprecedented in Israel: during the 42 days of Operation Desert Storm (16 January–25 February), Iraq fired 39 Scud missiles at Israel—initially suspected of carrying chemical warheads—on a total of 18 occasions. The extent of physical injuries caused by the attacks proved to be smaller than could be expected from the scope of the threat: two people were killed by direct missile hits, seven suffocated because of incorrect use of their gas masks, and four died of heart attacks caused by air raid sirens.[2] Nonetheless, the number of injured civilians was much greater than the small death toll would suggest. Israeli hospitals treated 1,059 patients in the wake of the attacks, over half of whom (544) suffered from symptoms of acute psychological stress (Solomon 1995). The acute stress reactions (ASR) were triggered primarily by the first missile attacks, which overturned expectations that Israel would be spared any bombardments, and that even if missiles were fired at Israel they would cause no damage. Even those who did not experience full-fledged acute stress reactions suffered the emotional stress caused by fears of a chemical attack on civilians. For example, 18% of those included in a sample of adults in attack-prone areas reported smelling gas during the missile bombardments. Most of the studies conducted during the war reported a significant rise in levels of anxiety, stress, fatigue, insomnia, concerns about failing to hear the siren, somatic complaints, and burnout (Milgram 1994).

The Gulf War placed the Israeli public face-to-face not only with its traumatic past but also with preconceptions about individual and collective strength and weakness. On the individual plane, the war constituted the first public reckoning with ASR, whose symptoms resemble those of CSR in soldiers. However, while the latter disorder had already been recognized by the Israel Defense Forces (IDF), ASR in civilians had yet to be known in Israel other than in singular cases in which personal weakness was thought to play a role. From a collective perspective, such incidents of acute stress triggered public consternation and alarm, which in turn produced contradictory attitudes toward ASR sufferers, and in extreme instances, even condemnation of acute stress sufferers for having succumbed to their fears. Although experts and official spokespersons encouraged the public to identify acute stress symptoms and alleviate them through self-help techniques or with the aid of professionals, civilians who relocated outside of the danger zones were harshly criticized, not only by court of public opinion but also by Israeli leaders. For example, Tel Aviv Mayor Shlomo Lahat called those who left the area "deserters," adding that "those who desert Tel Aviv also desert the homeland" ("Gulf War in Tel Aviv" 1991; Rice 2003). Lahat said out loud what many were thinking, prompting a ubiquity of pins and stickers bearing slogans such as "I'm a Tel Aviv patriot," which by implication denounced those who left Tel Aviv as "nonpatriots." Lahat's statement reflected the fear that panic would spread and the Israeli public's fortitude would crumble. However, linking patriotism with the decision to remain in a bombarded city lacking adequate defenses, with no clear advantage to the country's security, delegitimized fear as a reasonable response, and effectively assigned the responsibility for collective resilience to the individual. This dilemma between individual and national interests reflects the internal contradictions that characterize Israeli society's attitudes toward the interdependence of national and personal resilience, and the social meaning of war trauma. As awareness grew of acute stress reactions among civilians on the home front, and emphasized the cost of civilian sacrifice for national defense, this dilemma would come to preoccupy Israeli public discourse with greater intensity.

Concerns of a fear epidemic and impaired fortitude soon proved unfounded. On the whole, Israelis coped effectively with the emotional stresses of the war (Sheppard 2008). Starting with the second missile attack, a dramatic decline was registered in the number of acute stress sufferers, a decline that continued thereafter (Bleich et al. 1992). Even those diagnosed with ASR showed signs of recovery, although some 60% of them still had PTSD diagnoses one year later (Neria et al. 1998). In its 1991 annual national mood survey (conducted during the war), the Guttman Center found a slight (10%) decline in those who reported coping well with "the present situation," compared to the previous peacetime survey one year earlier.[3] Surprisingly, the percentage of respondents who reported a positive personal mood (75% of interviewees) increased from the previous year, a fact attributed by the authors of the survey to the psychological defense mechanism of self-reinforcement—a protective reaction against fundamental fear and anxiety. Moreover, civilians continued their routine: after the first four days of the Gulf War, most civilians returned to work, stores reopened, volunteers provided assistance to the elderly and to people with disabilities, and public institutions, including schools, reopened (Solomon 1995).

Noah Milgram, a renowned psychologist and expert on war-induced stress, attributed this resumption of normal activity to "adaption" and "habituation" behaviors. Civilians' adaptive behaviors included efforts to obtain information, use of hotlines to alleviate tension, and compliance with the instructions broadcast on the radio. Viewership of TV and radio programs featuring mental health experts soared. Habituation was reflected in a drastic decline in the number of calls made to the information, emergency, and assistance centers, and in the number of emergency patients hospitalized due to stress reactions or accidental auto-injection of atropine (a toxic material used to neutralize the effects of nerve gas that was disseminated to the population during the war). Milgram also notes that after the war there was a significant decrease in reports of psychological stress within the public at large, sometimes falling below prewar levels.

Therefore, the steep rise in the number of acute stress patients—overwhelming the capacity of the country's health care system—seems incongruous with the reports of high morale, volunteer activity, and absence of public panic.[4] However, such seemingly contradictory behavioral responses from a community in distress have been reported, in coexistence, in other, considerably more extreme historical situations. For example, both types of behaviors were observed simultaneously in the displaced persons (DP) camps in Germany, where Jews were concentrated after the Holocaust. Contemporaneous documents point to a kind of emotional dissonance among the survivors: obvious post-traumatic and depressive symptoms at the individual level, coupled with active, vibrant, diverse, and intensive communal life (Keynan 1996). While the two circumstances are fundamentally incomparable, these reports emphasize that even in events of major trauma, the community at large will often mobilize powers of resilience that enable it to cope as a group with the very conditions that challenge the fortitude of its individual members.

Communal adaptation may not only coincide with individual stress but also play an essential role in increasing individual resilience. Communal organizations, volunteer activity, and the perceived availability of "organizing forces" that provide guidance and assistance in times of distress all help build a support structure and contribute to its emotional and its instrumental effectiveness. As noted earlier (in Part I), lack of social support has been proven to be a risk factor for PTSD among combat soldiers. The same applies to civilians; social support improves their capacity to withstand situations that typically evoke traumatic stress (Bleich et al. 2003).

During the Gulf War, the media were awash in clinical discourse. In the first week of the war alone, 108 articles on mental health and another 72 articles and items dealing with psychological intervention were published in Israel's three major dailies (an average of ten items per day in each newspaper) (Milgram 1994).[5] This was no coincidence: the idea of an unconventional missile attack targeting civilians triggered a sense of helplessness previously unknown to Israelis. The helplessness intensified as the nation's leadership failed to convey that the situation was under control. Nearly the only audible authoritative voice at the time came from the IDF spokesperson who, in soothing tones, functioned as a buffer or shock absorber of the Scud attacks, instructing residents of targeted areas to enter or exit their sealed rooms, and explaining why they needed to wear their gas masks. An entire country hung on the words of the "national tranquillizer," as the IDF spokesperson became known, despite the limited range of solutions that he could offer. His legendary, oft-repeated instruction "Drink water" became a kind of cynical mantra in the Israeli lexicon (Lavie 2002).[6]

Forty percent of respondents to the Guttman Center wartime survey admitted feeling frightened and worried, while others dismissed possible traumatic psychological reactions to the war, and some objected to the very possibility of psychological traumatic reactions to the war. As the war continued, many op-eds deplored the fact that experts were repeatedly encouraging citizens to seek psychological help if needed. The authors argued that such encouragement implied the existence of a psychiatric disorder—an implication that they rejected all together. Even offers of assistance from mental health experts elicited mixed reactions. Forty percent of the respondents to a Dahaf Institute survey[7] conducted several months after the war reported that psychological counseling had helped them, particularly as it related to their children. These findings were offset, however, by critical, at times even cynical and derisive, warnings that referral to psychological aid was a pathetic response of authorities, who should have been preventing stress by resolving genuine concerns, such as inadequate public shelters. Even within the mental health community, criticism was directed at messages that allegedly focused on pathology rather than on normalcy, instead of proposing community-level support programs, which were underdeveloped at the time (Milgram 1994). While such criticism may have ultimately contributed to the development of community prevention and recovery intervention programs, during the Gulf War period such criticism represented a refusal to legitimize individual responses indicating weakness (Kimchi & Shamai 2006).

Strong traditional opposition of Israelis to legitimizing what they perceive as emotional weakness may also explain the government decision not to prepare the public for the war. Mental health experts criticized the political leadership for this decision, which was rooted in unjustified concerns that preparing the public for the crisis would cause even greater damage. In the critics' view, unpreparedness led to instances of needless atropine injection and to a loss of composure among a portion of the public (Shabtai Noy, quoted in Milgram 1994).

Despite the limited number of casualties, the Gulf War ultimately had profound ramifications for Israeli society. Holocaust survivors tended to experience higher levels of anxiety than other Israelis, even those of similar age, but all segments of the Israeli populace experienced a sense of helplessness and fear, and considered themselves victims of collective persecution (Solomon 1995). With the memory of Holocaust death camps a central motif in Israeli society, the threat of gas attacks awakened bitter associations. Although the government's decision to refrain from a military response garnered significant public support over the course of the war, some believed that the no-retaliation policy signaled weakness rather than restraint born of strength and fortitude.[8] The protection provided by sealed rooms seemed dubious, and the government-issued instructions were confusing, as one never knew whether the missiles being fired on the public carried conventional or chemical/biological warheads. Many thus detected a frightening similarity between the exilic Jewish history of passivity and powerlessness and the current strategy of restraint, which contrasted starkly with Israel's customarily assertive mode of response to threats since 1948.

The Gulf War also affected public confidence in the IDF's ability to defend the citizenry—whether because of the policy of restraint or the lack of technological means to prevent the missile attacks. For the first time in Israeli history, the IDF mounted no response to a security threat and failed to uphold one of the basic principles of its security doctrine: moving the war into enemy territory. The sense that Israel could not defend its citizenry from all threats, a disturbing idea in and of itself, became even more troubling when coupled with the general view that the country had been attacked despite having had no involvement in the events that led to the war. The frustration of having been attacked without provocation seemed to substantiate the societal belief that Israel was subject to persecution only because it was a Jewish state, reinforcing the existing Israeli mentality of victimization (Bar-Tal 1998).

The Gulf War also marked a disintegration of the relative sense of security of the home front and obscured the formerly clear division between home front and war front. In the new and menacing reality, the war front spread to the urban population centers and into the home; the casualties were mainly civilians, and the army had no solution. In this, the Gulf War prefigured the crisis triggered three years later by the terrorist attacks mounted in opposition to the Oslo Accords, and the wave of terrorism of the early 2000s.

Theoretically, this new reality should have challenged civilians' secondary status on the Israeli heroism scale. It was only during the latter half of the 1990s, however, and with even greater momentum in the early 2000s—two periods in which Israeli urban centers were subject to deadly terrorist attacks—that the demand for civilian victims of hostilities to be accorded equal status with soldiers burst onto the public agenda. Why was this demand not voiced during the Gulf War, when it was Israeli civilians alone who were under fire? One might postulate that the demand did not emerge at the time because most of the injured civilians, for whom such a demand was relevant, suffered from acute stress reaction. Psychological trauma is not an injury generally seen as having a heroic dimension; a war in which it constituted the main form of injury could not drive any change in the status of civilians within the hierarchy of heroism, despite the major role the victims played.

The Gulf War's impact should therefore be understood not necessarily through individual cases of psychological stress, but rather through its collective impact on the national mood, in the emergent consensus that Israel's military capabilities should be reinforced, and in a nascent familiarity with the broader phenomenon of individual war-related psychological trauma. The war reawakened preexisting fears of a *national trauma*—the kind that could strike a fatal blow to the entire national collective, and in the face of which the collective is completely helpless. In retrospect, however, the harm actually suffered by Israeli society during the Gulf War constituted *individual injury of war-induced trauma, due to national affiliation*. While civilians paid a heavy emotional and physical toll as a result of hostile activity that targeted their nation-state, the events themselves posed no existential threat to the collective.[9] Hence, the Gulf War's relevance for our discussion lies in its role as a watershed event that divided earlier conceptions of national trauma from a more sophisticated understanding of how national wars affect individuals, and the interdependence between the two concepts.

In retrospect, the Gulf War signaled a new era in the way Israelis perceived their security risks and the chances for regional peace. The unprovoked missile attacks targeting civilians, accompanied with threats of chemical warheads, had a profound and long-term impact on Israelis' collective consciousness. It reactivated the national trauma of the Holocaust and the national conviction that as a Jewish state, Israel will always be persecuted regardless of its policy. It undermined the collective sense of security under the protection of the IDF, and confronted society with the bloodless injury of PTSD, which in itself posed a threat to the national resilience. In the next round of violence, three years later, civilian trauma came to center stage, in a process that reached its peak in the Al-Aqsa Intifada during 2000–2004. The Gulf War and the subsequent terrorist attacks on the Israeli civilian public triggered a rethinking about civilian roles in war, and reinforced the protest against their lower rank on the heroism scale.

The Al-Aqsa Intifada: "Even the Numbers Are Traumatic"

October 2000 witnessed the eruption of the Second, or Al-Aqsa, Intifada, which was to last for four years. In that span, 743 hostile acts were perpetrated in civilian population centers, killing 719 Israelis and wounding 6,862 (Baer 2007).[10] The terrorist attacks affected not only the victims but also Israeli society as a whole. In 2003, 16.4% of all Israelis reported having personally experienced a terror attack and an additional 40% reported that a family member or friend had the experience (Bleich et al. 2003).[11] The circle of bereavement also expanded profoundly: a 2004 study found that over a fifth of Israelis had lost relatives or friends during the Intifada.[12] In other words, every sixth civilian had directly encountered terrorism, every fifth citizen had lost someone close, and nearly one in every three citizens had a relative or friend who had experienced a terrorist attack.

The attacks' pervasive ripple effect, and their high frequency, disrupted the fabric of Israeli life, particularly during the first two and a half years of the Intifada, when terrorist attacks were particularly frequent (60 suicide attacks were committed in 2002 alone; Israel Intelligence Heritage and Commemoration Center 2005).[13] The knowledge that an attack could occur virtually anywhere, at any given moment, had a destructive impact on everyday civilian habits. People felt a constant need to know where their family members and close friends were at all times, and confined their activities to areas that seemed safe. Over half of the respondents to a 2002 Dahaf Institute survey reported a significant decline in their ventures outside the home, and half of this group reported a very sharp decline (i.e., to the point of hardly ever leaving their homes). This situation affected the overall national mood and, in turn, the economy. Leisure and hospitality industries were virtually paralyzed, as indicated by the record low in Israel's annual figures for hotel occupancy.[14] The economic recession exacerbated the population's sense of insecurity.[15] For two consecutive years (2001 and 2002), Israel recorded a real decline in GDP, and unemployment rose to 10.9% by the final quarter of 2003.[16]

Trauma researchers argue that the Second Intifada's extraordinary impact on the public was due to the particular nature of terrorist attacks: they were sudden and overwhelming, and one couldn't know how to avoid them (Somer & Bleich 2005). Studies have shown that, in contrast to the trauma caused by natural and technological disasters, the trauma induced by terrorist attacks is particularly profound (Tuval-Mashiah & Shalev 2005). Such attacks undermine an individual's basic assumptions about safety in her environment, residence, and everyday life, and give rise to severe adjustment difficulties. The attacks occur repeatedly yet randomly—they frustrate individuals' attempts to develop a forecasting model or to determine the most effective means of avoiding them in the course of one's daily activities (ibid.). Trauma of this kind, referred to in the literature as Type-IV Stress, is produced by exposure to exceptionally threatening and shocking scenes, and by the knowledge that the same traumatic elements are likely to recur at an unknown time and place.[17]

These conditions gave rise to an especially high rate of acute stress within the civilian population. In October 2003, the Ministry of Health (MOH) estimated that as many as 1,300 individuals suffered from emotional trauma. A year and a half later, MOH figures indicated that between 2,800 and 3,000 people (40%–50% of all those wounded in the Intifada) suffered acute stress at various levels of severity (Marciano & Meir 2005).[18]

Meanwhile, post-traumatic symptoms were also reported by a significant number of civilians indirectly affected by terrorism. Of the numerous studies and surveys published during the Intifada period on the effects of violence on Israeli society, and looking at society as a whole—those who were directly exposed to terror and those who were not—nearly all indicated widespread fear and ASR within the population. A 2002 telephone survey of 512 households, constituting a representative sample of the Israeli population, found that 76.7% of the respondents experienced at least one PTSD symptom (Bleich et al. 2003). According to a series of studies on the varying levels of injury within the public at large, 4.4% were afflicted with full-blown PTSD (measured using conservative criteria) while 25% reported moderate symptoms of PTSD. The most prevalent symptoms were intrusive memories of the event, even if viewed in the media, recurring flashbacks, and a deep sense of sadness and grief (Tuval-Mashiah & Shalev 2005).

Other research showed that a significant proportion of the population experienced a threat to their lives and the lives of their loved ones (60.5% and 67.9%, respectively); respondents also reported high levels of tension (54%) and moderate (58.6%) and high (30%) levels of sadness (Bleich et al. 2003; Tuval-Mashiah & Shalev 2005). In response to a May 2003 Guttman Center survey, 83% of the respondents stated that they were worried or very worried (40%) that they or members of their families might be injured in a terrorist incident. For purposes of comparison, the last figure is nearly four times higher than its parallel from January 1999.[19]

The National Security Studies Center at the University of Haifa has been conducting a continuous valuation of levels of fear and endurance within the Israeli populace since 2000 (Ben-Dor 2003). The assessment uses a series of items, rated by respondents on a scale from 1 to 6, intended to gauge levels of fear in four categories: fear of terrorism affecting the respondent and his family, fear of terrorism affecting everyday life, terrorism as a strategic danger to Israel, and fear of an attack disrupting the political system. During the Intifada, fear levels on all four categories ranged from 4.91 to 5.19 (Ben-Dor et al. 2006).[20] The researchers noted that this is the highest level of fear ever measured in the Western world, with the exception of the ten days subsequent to the 9/11 attacks.

The emotional status of children was another cause for concern. In 2003, 9% of Israeli children reported clinically significant PTSD symptoms, while an additional 15% reported symptoms ranging from moderate to very severe. These figures may have been underestimated. In the study submitted to the Committee on the Status of Children of the Israeli Parliament by Dr. Avital Lauder of Tel Aviv University, the most worrisome conclusion was that 42% of all children reported moderate to very severe symptoms.[21] Significantly, the study found no direct connection between PTSD symptomology, place of residence, and direct exposure to terrorism.

Laufer and Solomon showed that fear, as a subjective perception of threat, is the variable most closely correlated with PTSD symptoms, outweighing place of residence and even objective exposure to terrorism.[22] American studies conducted in the wake of 9/11 yielded similar findings, as did other Israeli studies (Cohen Silver et al. 2002). These findings assume special significance in view of the country's small size, where geographic proximity and personal relations connect large proportions of society to any given event, and exacerbate individuals' perceived proximity to each attack. This, in turn, creates a pervasive sense of danger and a dismal national mood.

Massive media coverage made things seem even bleaker. As in the Gulf War, during the Al-Aqsa Intifada, the Israeli media quoted extensively from studies and surveys. The abundance of new media outlets and the duration of the Intifada amplified the coverage of civilian trauma. For example, my search of the influential daily *Haaretz* in March 2003—a month chosen at random—yields 59 articles, nearly 2 per day, devoted to issues of terrorism-related trauma or ASR, 39 of which specifically referred to the Intifada. My Google search produced 1,260 Hebrew links to items related to the Intifada and ASR, and 750 images of trauma sufferers, or nearly one textual link per day (1.15) and an image every second day (1.94) over the four-year period of the Intifada. These figures are comparable to 100 articles and almost 100 images per day, over four years, in a population the size of the US: a random search in the *New York Times* (equivalent to Israel's *Haaretz*) between September 11, 2001, and October 10, 2001, retrieved only 31 articles.

The full range of news items and articles is too great to be described here, but it is crucial to note that most of them were accompanied by disturbing, even harrowing headlines. For example, one article reported that 60% of children aged ten and under in the settlement of Psagot suffered from urinary incontinence (*Shavu'on Yerushalayim*, April 19, 2001). Another, entitled "A Traumatized City," reported study findings to the effect that one in eight children in Jerusalem displayed PTSD symptoms (*Shavu'on Yerushalayim*, July 5, 2002). One article declared, in bold type, that "we are a depressed people" looking for someone to turn to for help (Moscona-Lerman 2002). And another claimed, "We don't even have someone to complain to" (Firkash 2003). The newspaper articles, and especially their sensational headlines, added force to the findings, often presenting them in an exaggerated light. For example, one major April 2003 article, reporting on the aforementioned Solomon and Laufer study, proclaimed that 42% of Israeli children, regardless of their place of residence, suffered from "shock" (Eldar 2003). A careful reading, however, reveals that only 9% of the children in the study reported post-traumatic symptoms of clinical significance, while others reported symptoms at varying levels that did not imply a PTSD diagnosis. In other words, public levels of anxiety in Israel, high to begin with, were further elevated by data presented injudiciously and with insufficient explanation to an audience lacking the expertise to understand them properly. Ultimately, media reporting itself was often considered a threat to public fortitude: reported Israeli PTSD figures were so high that it seemed that "even the numbers [were] traumatic" (Arad 2003).

Not all the study and survey findings could be taken at face value. A portion of the findings focused on respondent feelings, with no attention to functional impairment; others were obtained via telephone surveys, whose reliability is lower than that of face-to-face interviews (Cohen & Yahav 2010). Most of the findings included post-traumatic symptoms of varying severity levels, regardless of whether they constituted full-blown PTSD, and included no attempt to assess the correlation or continuity between the various criteria—one of the litmus tests in diagnosing PTSD (Young 2007). Diverse diagnostic and measurement methods also make it hard to compare the data yielded by the various studies. Nevertheless, the findings were significant in directing public attention to terror-related trauma, as a result of which terror-related trauma became a legitimate topic of debate, beginning to influence Ministry of Health and National Insurance Institute decisions concerning the care of the emotionally traumatized.

The general public mood remained gloomy, despite other, more reassuring voices of encouragement ("We overcame Pharaoh, we'll get through this as well")[23] and displays of strength and determination ("Hadera, After Nine Fatalities: We Won't Buckle"; Ratner 2002). This inundation of trauma discourse encountered opponents who feared the impact of a drastic transition from a national ethos of a nation whose sons "do not cry" to an excessive discourse of emotional trauma. The objectors feared that the trauma discourse would prompt a national climate of victimization, and that the enemy would disrupt the normal course of Israeli life by targeting the country's "soft underbelly"—its new sensitivity to the emotional status of civilians.[24] Public attention was increasingly drawn to the strategic impact of openly expressed anxiety, which was frequently interpreted as panic or hysteria (Ringel-Hoffman 2001), which—they feared—would create some truth in Hassan Nasrallah's October 2000 pronouncement: "Israel has nuclear weapons and the strongest air force in the region, but the truth is that it is weaker than a spider's web."[25]

Notes

1. The author explains that assertiveness and activity in self-defense are crucial to Israelis' sense of security.
2. In addition, the number of deaths for cardiac reasons increased in the first days, especially in Tel Aviv and Haifa, regions heavily struck by missiles (Sheppard 2008).
3. The Guttman Institute for Applied Social Research conducts an annual survey of the Israeli national mood from various perspectives (henceforth "Guttman Center"). The component survey in question was conducted by Shlomit Levy. During periods of calm the usual percentage of those reporting positive personal mood ranges from 60% to 70%. Data per Milgram (1994, p. 9). The Guttman Center became part of the Israeli Democracy Institute in 1998, and all the survey data, including from pre-1998 years, are available at www.idi.org.il.
4. See the review of a series of studies on this topic in Milgram (1994).
5. It is important to note that for a country of the size of Israel, this is a huge number of articles.
6. Lavie bases his article on an unpublished study conducted by Major Uriel Ben-Ami for the IDF History Department.
7. Dahaf Institute is a leading public survey institute.
8. This support ranged from 80% just prior to the missile attacks to 70% during the first week of the war, rising again to 80% during the middle of the war's second week, after the population had adjusted to the situation (Milgram 1994, p. 8).
9. On the difference between individual and collective trauma, see Neal (1998).
10. The data refer to the period from the start of the Intifada (28 September 2000) to the end of 2004 (the Intifada's end date is a matter of dispute; in this book I place it at the end of 2004). Israeli Foreign Ministry data indicate that 132 of the incidents were suicide attacks, in which 502 people lost their lives (retrieved 1 February 2010 from the Foreign Ministry website: www.mfa.gov.il/MFA). Per B'Tselem data, 3,113 Palestinians were killed during the same period (retrieved 20 June 2010 from the B'Tselem website: www.btselem.org/Hebrew). See also the introduction in Somer and Bleich (2005). These figures do not include the rocket attacks on Sderot and southern Israel. The number of hostile events counted by the National Insurance Institute includes all incidents designated as hostile events by the Approving Authority during the period in question. The Approving Authority is a committee appointed by the minister of defense in consultation with the minister of social affairs; it is authorized to determine that a given event is indeed a "hostile act." On this topic see Rimmerman et al. (2007).
11. The exact figure is 37.3%.
12. The precise figure was 21.8% (Ben-Dor et al. 2006).
13. In 2001 there were 35 suicide attacks; the peak of 60 in 2002 was followed by a drastic decline to 26 in 2003 and to 13 in 2004.
14. Occupancy was 38.8% versus 54.4% in 1999 (Data of the Central Bureau of Statistics, retrieved 1 February 2010 from: www.cbs.gov.il/ts/IDb609046ddd0f6e [Hebrew]). A decline in the number of tourists also affected the hotel occupancy rate.

15. In 2002 only 39.5% of respondents to the Central Bureau of Statistics Social Survey expected their economic status to improve in the coming years, versus 45.2% in, for instance, 2007. Respectively, 48% responded in 2002 that they were satisfied with their economic status, compared with 53.1% in 2007. In September 2004 28.8% of Israelis reported that the Intifada had caused them financial loss (Ben-Dor et al., 2004).
16. In 2002, GDP declined by 3.1%, after a similar drop in 2001. The year 2003 witnessed a turnaround: GDP rose by 1.3% (Bank of Israel Annual Report 2003, retrieved 1 February 2010 from: www.bankisrael.org.il/deptdata/mehkar/doch03/heb/p_nagid.htm). The unemployment data are also from the Bank of Israel website (Statistical Supplement to the Bank of Israel Annual Report 2003, retrieved 20 June 2010 [Hebrew]).
17. "Type IV Stress" is defined by J. P. Wilson 1994, 'The Need for an Integrative Theory of Post-Traumatic Stress Disorder' in *Handbook of Post Traumatic Theory*, eds. M. B. Williams & J. F. Sommer, Jr., Greenwood, Westport, CT, quoted in Somer and Bleich (2005).
18. The authors use Ministry of Health data.
19. Guttman Center. From the Israel Democracy Institute database (henceforth "Guttman Center"): National Security and Public Opinion, January 1999, February 1997, Elections Study, May 1996, Elections Study, January 2003. [Hebrew]
20. The sample includes Jews and non-Jews.
21. Solomon and Laufer, quoted in Caspi (2003); also see Israel, Knesset (2003).
22. Quoted in Caspi (2003).
23. The city of Hadera, established in 1891, is located about 28 miles north of Tel Aviv. N. Nevet 2003, At [women's magazine], April; see also Z. Cohen 2002, "Have We Really Grown Used to Terrorism?" *Yedioth Ahronoth*. 19 June. [Hebrew]
24. Confidential testimonies, NATAL Documentation Department, Testimony NT/AT.
25. Statement of Nasrallah on 26 May 2000, quoted in "'National Resilience': Victory on the Home Front—a Conceptual Framework," document submitted by the Reut Institute to the Knesset Foreign Affairs and Defense Committee's Subcommittee on Home-Front Readiness, headed by MK Ami Ayalon, November 2008 (henceforth "National Resilience"). Retrieved 25 August 2009 from: http://reut-institute.org/Publication.aspx?PublicationID=3487. [English version: http://reut-institute.org/Publication.aspx?PublicationId=3488]

References

Arad, T. 2003, 'Terrorism's Emotional Damage: Even the Numbers Are Traumatic', *Iton Yerushalayim*, 25 April. (Hebrew)

Baer, S. 2007, *Recipients of Hostile Acts Benefits, 2006*, National Insurance Institute, Research and Planning Administration. Available from www.btl.gov.il/Publications/survey%5CPages/Seker212.aspx.

Bar-Tal, D. 1998, 'Societal Beliefs in Times of Intractable Conflict: the Israeli Case', *International Journal of Conflict Management, 1997–2002*, vol. 9, no. 1, pp. 22–50.

Ben-Dor, G. 2003, 'The "Haifa Indicators": Report of a Cross-Functional Team'. Paper presented at the Fourth Herzliya Conference, Herzliya. Available from www.herzliyaconference.org/_Uploads/1028gabibendor.pdf [31 January 2010]. (Hebrew)

Ben-Dor, G., Canetti, D., & Halperin, E. 2006, 'The Social Component of National Resilience', presentation given at the Sixth Herzliya Conference, Herzliya. Available from www.herzliyaconference.org/_Uploads/2131hosen_heb.pdf [30 January 2010]. (Hebrew)

Ben-Dor, G., Pedahzur, A., & Canetti, D. 2004, 'The Social Component of National Resilience', presentation given at the Herzliya Conference, Herzliya. Available from www.herzliyaconference.org/_Uploads/1794madHaifa1.pdf [31 January 2010]. (Hebrew)

Bleich, A., Dycian, A., Koslovsky, M., Solomon, Z., & Weiner, M. 1992, 'Psychiatric Implications of Missile Attacks on a Civilian Population', *Journal of the American Medical Association*, vol. 268, pp. 613–615.

Bleich, A., Gelkopf, M., & Solomon, Z. 2003, 'Exposure to Terrorism, Stress-Related Mental Health Symptoms, and Coping Behaviors among a Nationally Representative Sample in Israel', *JAMA*, vol. 290, pp. 612–620.

Caspi, M. 2003, Research and Information Center, the Knesset, background document for deliberations on the topic of terrorism-related anxiety among children. Available from www.knesset.gov.il/mmm/data/pdf/m00608.pdf.

Cohen, M., & Yahav, R. 2010, 'Stress Reactions among Residents of Northern and Central Israel and among Jews and Arabs during the Second Lebanon War' in *Health, Education and Welfare Services in Times of Crisis: Lessons Learned from the Second Lebanon War*, eds. F. Azaiza, N. Nachmias, & M. Cohen, Pardes, Haifa, pp. 77–93. (Hebrew)

Cohen Silver, R., Holman, A. E., McIntosh, D. N., Poulin, M., & Gil-Rivas, V. 2002, 'Nationwide Longitudinal Study of Psychological Responses to September 11', *JAMA*, vol. 288, pp. 1235–1244.

Eldar, A. 2003, 'Four of Every Ten Israeli Children Suffering from PTSD', *Haaretz*, 24 April. (Hebrew)

Firkash, T. 2003, '40% of Children Suffering Anxiety Due to the Terrorist Attacks', *HaTzofe*, 10 October. (Hebrew)

'The Gulf War in Tel Aviv' 1991, Tel Aviv-Jaffa Municipality. Available from http://tel-aviv.millenium.org.il/NR/exeres/6F3B8AFC-6AB0–47AC-A624-E72CDE059538,frameless.htm [13 June 2009].

Israel, Knesset 2003, minutes, no. 3, 4 June.

Israel Intelligence Heritage and Commemoration Center 2005, 'Five Years since the Outbreak of the Violent Confrontation between Israel and the Palestinians: Features and Data'. Available from www.terrorism-info.org.il/malam_multimedia/Hebrew/heb_n/pdf/con_5y.pdf [1 February 2014].

Keynan, I. 1996, *The Hunger Has Not Abated, Holocaust Survivors and the Emissaries from Eretz Israel, Germany 1945–1948*, Am Oved, Tel Aviv.

Kimchi, S., & Shamai, M. 2006, 'Community Resilience as a Buffer of Stress Reactions', *Social Issues in Israel*, vol. 1, pp. 152–170. (Hebrew)

Lavie, A. 2002, 'Nachman, the Next War, and Me', *Walla! Hadashot*, 2 October.

Lazarus, R. S. 1986, 'The Psychology of Stress and Coping' in *Stress and Anxiety*, vol. 10, eds. C. D. Spielberger & I. C. Sarason, Hemisphere, Washington D.C., pp. 399–418.

Marciano, I., & Meir, O. 2005, 'Since the Start of the Intifada, Thousands Suffer Trauma', *Ynet*, 5 January. (Hebrew)

Milgram, N. 1994, 'Psychological Research in Israel during the Gulf War', *Psikhologia*, vol. 4, no. 1–2, pp. 7–19. (Hebrew)

Moscona-Lerman, B. 2002, *Maariv*, Holiday Magazine, 2 April. (Hebrew)

Neal, A. G. 1998, *National Trauma and Collective Memory: Major Events in the American Century*, M E Sharpe, Armonk, NY.

Neria, Y., Solomon, Z., Ginzburg, K., Dekel, R., Enoch, D., & Ohry, A. 1998, 'Wars and Their Psychological Cost: Aspects of Psychological Trauma among Soldiers and Civilians in Israeli Society', *Society and Welfare*, vol. 18, no. 1, pp. 125–139.

Ratner, D. 2002, 'Hadera, after Nine Fatalities: We Won't Buckle', *Haaretz*, 6 June.

Rice, O. 2003, 'Gentlemen, History Is Repeating Itself', *Ynet*, 18 March. (Hebrew)

Rimmerman, A., Tal-Katz, P., & Avrami, S. 2007, 'People Injured in Acts of Terror in Israel and the United States: a Comparative Review and Future Recommendations', *Social Security*, vol. 73, pp. 41–68. (Hebrew)

Ringel-Hoffman, A. 2001, 'Terrorism's Triumph Lies in the Panic It Creates', *Yedioth Ahronoth, Saturday Supplement*, 9 March. (Hebrew)

Sheppard, B. 2008, *The Psychology of Strategic Terrorism: Public and Government Responses to Attack*, Routledge, New York.

Solomon, Z. 1995, *Coping with War-Induced Stress: the Gulf War and the Israeli Response*, Plenum Press, New York.

Somer, E., & Bleich, A. 2005, 'Stress in a Population under Prolonged Terrorist Attack: Identification, Characterization and Treatment Challenges' in *Mental Health in Terror's Shadow: the Israeli Experience*, eds. E. Somer & A. Bleich, Ramot, Tel Aviv. (Hebrew)

Tuval-Mashiah, R., & Shalev, A. 2005, 'The Epidemiology of Mental Responses to Continuous Terrorism among Adults in Israel' in *Mental Health in Terror's Shadow: the Israeli Experience*, eds. E. Somer & A. Bleich, Ramot, Tel Aviv, pp. 29–54. (Hebrew)

Wilson, J. P. 1994, 'The Need for an Integrative Theory of Post-Traumatic Stress Disorder', in *Handbook of Post Traumatic Theory*, eds. M. B. Williams & J. F. Sommer, Jr., Greenwood, Westport, CT, pp. 3–18.

Young, A. 2007, '9/11: Mental Health in the Wake of Terrorist Attacks', *Journal of Nervous and Mental Disease*, vol. 195, no. 12, p. 1030.

9 From Denial to Recognition

Trauma Discourse on the Public Agenda

The Al-Aqsa Intifada[1] placed individual psychological war-related trauma at the center of Israeli public discourse, where it has remained ever since. The wave of terrorism collectively known as the Al-Aqsa Intifada occurred nearly two decades after the attitudes toward soldiers suffering combat stress reaction (CSR) and PTSD showed the first indications of change. The medical establishment had gradually come to realize that its longtime disregard of these phenomena had been a "historical professional mistake" (Levy et al. 1990), which it was determined not to repeat. This new approach trickled down to the general public as well, in part due to the actions of civil society and self-help organizations, as well as the 2000 decision of the National Insurance Institute (NII) to recognize PTSD for disability-rating purposes.[2]

The beginning of the third millennium has also witnessed a wave of terrorism outside Israel, the most notable instance of which is 9/11. This catastrophe, which cost the lives of 2,976 people,[3] had an impact not only on American society and politics but also on air travel and on attitudes toward terrorism throughout the Western world. One outcome of the event was the spotlight it directed to PTSD in public and scientific circles, both in the US and elsewhere. The fact that the Al-Aqsa Intifada and 9/11 occurred at around the same time reinforced the Israeli media and the public preoccupation with terrorism and its effects, increasingly including the immediate and long-term traumatic reactions experienced by victims and witnesses. According to Criterion A1 for PTSD in the 1994 edition of the APA's *Diagnostic and Statistical Manual of Mental Disorders* (DSM-IV), a person is said to suffer from PTSD if she was exposed to a threat of death or serious injury, or witnessed such a threat to others, and experienced a strong emotional reaction to the event, characterized by fear, helplessness, or horror. This definition was modified in the 2013 DSM-V (APA 2013), and excluded distant and media exposure,[4] but at the time of 9/11 and Al-Aqsa Intifada, the DSM definition also acknowledged the destructive impact of indirect exposure to a traumatic event, even if the affected person was not on the scene. Despite the argument mounted by some professionals that this inclusion constituted an exaggerated clinical interpretation of the PTSD diagnostic criteria, indirect exposure as a criterion was retained in the DSM-IV's "text revision" published in 2000.[5] This definition made it possible to acknowledge the causal link between a terrorist event and a traumatic injury, even if exposure took place via the media. Against this background, an exceedingly high prevalence of post-traumatic symptoms was found among American citizens in the aftermath of 9/11. In a nationwide study conducted several days after the catastrophe, 44% of American adults reported one or more symptoms of major stress (Schuster et al. 2001). Another study, conducted five to eight weeks later, found that 7.5% of all Manhattan residents and 20% of all residents of the area surrounding the World Trade Center were experiencing symptoms consistent with the PTSD definition (Galea et al. 2002). Although some scholars did not find indirect exposure to the Twin Towers bombing by itself to be related to PTSD (Neria et al. 2006), there have been several studies in post-9/11 national samples that provided evidence of the possibility of such connection.

These findings—which are similar to Israeli findings of PTSD prevalence—reinforced the criticism of the expansive PTSD definition, even giving rise to claims that trauma discourse had moved from one extreme—denial—to another—exaggeration. I will address the validity of these claims in the concluding part of the book (Part III); in any case, there can be no doubt that the trauma discourse triggered by early twenty-first-century terrorism unquestionably constituted a turning point, after which civilian war-related emotional trauma could no longer be swept under the rug.

In Israel, the Al-Aqsa Intifada and the 1973 Yom Kippur War had a special effect on the acknowledgment of war trauma. Both events managed to dispel the traditional "episodic amnesia"[6] that had previously caused the "disappearance" of accumulated data on war trauma. This pattern of "forgetfulness," which had prevailed both internationally and in Israel with regard to CSR and PTSD, also prevailed in Israel regarding civilian acute stress reactions (ASR). Accordingly, the scholarly and journalistic coverage of ASR, which made intensive headway into the public consciousness during the Gulf War and for some time afterward, gradually dissipated, all but forgotten. Three years after that war, no systematic epidemiological data on the distribution of PTSD among Israeli civilians were being collected (Regulant-Levy 1994). And yet, just as the Yom Kippur War had put an end to the former sweeping denial of combat stress, the Al-Aqsa Intifada similarly halted the cycle of oblivion with regard to civilian war trauma, and altered public attitudes to the present.

It seems that just as the Yom Kippur War directed public attention to the suffering of the individual soldier on the battlefield, the Al-Aqsa Intifada was the main catalyst for attitudinal change toward the personal suffering of civilians—as victims of terrorist events or their family members.

There were, however, many significant differences between the Yom Kippur War and the Al-Aqsa Intifada. The Yom Kippur War was an existential war that endangered the very existence of Israel. The threat represented by the Al-Aqsa Intifada, however, despite its large death and injury toll, was more limited in terms of the existence of Israel. As agonizing and intolerable as it was, Israel's existence was not at risk. Nonetheless, the Intifada resembled the Gulf War, in that both events were situated on the seam line between collective trauma suffered by the nation and trauma suffered by individuals on account of their nationality. In both events, Israelis felt the threat of a shared disaster, but in neither case was the collective's future actually at risk; it was the physical and emotional integrity of its individual members that was under threat.

Still, the Al-Aqsa Intifada was unique in the frequency with which physical and psychological injuries occurred, its duration, and the number of individuals who sustained injury. These statistics represented a critical mass that made it impossible to continue suppressing the price paid by civilians in war, of which emotional trauma is a part, and created a climate that facilitated challenges to civilians' secondary status on the heroism and bereavement scale. At the same time, the figures conveyed that acute stress reactions to hostile acts, just as physical injuries, are not random or tragic workings of fate, but rather the personal price that the individual pays as a member of the nation.

Discourse and Reality: The Governmental Establishment

Prior to the late twentieth century, no Israeli legislation addressed the issue of civilians afflicted with war trauma: the matter is not mentioned in the Compensation for Victims of Hostile Acts Law 5730–1970, which remains the basis for eligibility of victims of hostile acts for assistance. In this period, the needs of the psychologically injured were only incompletely addressed by the NII, the entity responsible for implementing the law and the sole authority to determine eligibility for benefits. Based on a 1988 amendment to the law, where it was hinted that mental impairment could be a form of recognizable disability,[7] limited cases were recognized, where officials felt that they had "sufficient" information to make such determination.[8]

The first meaningful change in NII's policy on acute stress reaction (ASR) casualties occurred in 2000. In October of that year, the NII added a section on PTSD to its disability rating tests (Yanay et al. 2005). This was an administrative order, not legislation, but it did have important practical implications. Although it entitled PTSD sufferers a disability rating of only 9%, which is too low to be of much use in securing adequate monetary compensation for the effects of trauma, it significantly increased the number of those recognized as disabled on the basis of this addition (ibid.). Six years later, based on the experience of the Second Lebanon War (2006) and due to the large number of people traumatized by that war, the services for casualties of psychological trauma were separated from services oriented toward the needs of the physically injured, and a national hotline was established for this purpose. The hotline was formally intended for ASR sufferers treated at hospitals in the wake of hostile acts, but even the non-hospitalized injured were able to get through since the system did not require identification (Baer 2007). Moreover, the Ministry of Social Affairs, in cooperation with the Ministry of Health, established resilience and community stress prevention centers (resilience centers), whose goal was to improve the coping skills of individuals and communities facing emergency situations and experiencing acute stress reactions.[9]

This important advance notwithstanding, scholars note that it is very difficult to obtain NII recognition as the victim of a hostile act on the basis of PTSD (Rimmerman et al. 2007). This argument is supported by testimonies of trauma sufferers who describe the enormous difficulty of interacting with the NII, which they at times characterize as displaying an abusive attitude.[10] The problems they encounter include attempts by medical committees to trace the source of trauma to a previous psychological disturbance, and excessive bureaucratic red tape, in which many applicants are unable to document precisely the incidents in which they were injured or prove that their injury was caused by one of a list of "approved" events.[11] The obstacles that such documentation requirements pose are especially relevant for individuals traumatized by events whose temporal boundaries are unclear, such as missile bombardments that took place over a period of time (sometimes months or even years) or a series of terrorist attacks. In places such as Sderot,[12] which are subject to repeated rocket attacks over years, and in areas that have been exposed repeatedly to terrorism, such as Jerusalem and Tel Aviv during the Al-Aqsa Intifada, documenting the exact incidents that triggered traumatic reactions is an unsurpassable challenge for most acute stress and PTSD casualties.

Researchers, NII personnel, and the Terror Victims [Representative] Association (the Association) concur that the arduous NII process deters many trauma casualties from even filing a claim (Rimmerman et al. 2007). In an article in the Association's newsletter *HaTikva* during the Second Lebanon War, the Association's then-director Menashe Pur-David maintained that thousands of ASR sufferers had not been officially recognized as victims of hostilities, due to the insurmountable obstacles piled by NII on those seeking to prove their psychological damage and that it had been directly caused by a hostile act. Many trauma casualties, according to Pur-David, "after failing again and again to prove their distress to the establishment, simply gave up."[13] Rimmerman et al. (2007) suggest that those who sustain psychological trauma and never seek compensation from the NII are liable to live in the shadow of the traumatizing event all their lives.

The NII offers 12 sessions of psychological counseling to trauma sufferers who have either filed a claim or undergone treatment in a hospital or a resilience center. In practice, however, the right to counseling turns out to be conditional and awarded in only certain instances. According to the NII website, NII-funded psychotherapy is available only to people whose disabilities impair their everyday functioning, and even then, only when rehabilitation personnel affirm that "therapy of this kind may improve [the claimant's] emotional and mental status and aid in the rehabilitation of the acute stress sufferer."[14] This criterion reflects the narrow, employment-focused rehabilitation approach shared by the NII and the Ministry of Defense, and runs counter to the already well-known fact, noted in the introduction to this volume, that many trauma sufferers manage to function well at work but experience serious emotional problems that profoundly affect their quality of life and often irreversibly compromise their social-familial relationships. Many of these people need not only rehabilitation as understood by the NII but also emotional assistance to alleviate the impact of trauma on their social interactions and everyday lives. Restricted access to psychological counseling leaves many of these trauma sufferers unserved, and in fact many PTSD sufferers consequently turn to volunteer organizations for assistance.

The importance of access to psychological treatment is underscored by studies pointing to higher recovery rates when intervention takes place at early stages (Somer & Bleich 2005). In practice, however, only a minority of trauma casualties actually seek counseling. The study by Bleich et al. (2003) quoted earlier (see Chapter 8) found that 76.7% of the respondents suffered from at least one symptom of PTSD, yet only 5.3% of them had sought psychological aid. While these data may reflect the common Israeli aversion to psychotherapy, they may also reflect the difficulties experienced by traumatized people in access to such treatment. The aforementioned study also found that 12.2% had called public hotlines, which may reflect the difference between acute need for help in an emergency and a long-term commitment to psychological treatment, but it also indicates the importance of easy and quick access to professional help. In confidential testimonies I collected during the 2012 and 2014 wars in Gaza, the interviewees—all with reactivated war trauma—were reluctant to obtain the therapy they needed. Their reluctance was based on the difficulty of finding a suitable therapist, and because it seemed an admission of the weakness they were trying to hide. The hotlines, on the other hand, seemed to them a reasonable, accessible solution.[15]

Findings of a comprehensive study conducted in the US between 1995 and 2000 (Kessler 2000) similarly found that only one-third of those diagnosed with PTSD in a nationwide survey were currently in therapy. A significant proportion of the untreated respondents did recognize the need for therapy; the most prevalent reason they gave for not being treated was lack of access, lack of financial resources to pay for counseling, or lack of information on how and where to obtain therapy. The study authors note that not only do states and the federal governments have a moral obligation to create the conditions for care, but also they actually have good economic reasons to encourage as many trauma sufferers as possible to seek counseling without delay. Untreated trauma sufferers often have trouble keeping jobs, and they develop physical ailments more frequently than others, meaning that they and their families need more services from the state. The cost of aiding citizens whose trauma goes untreated greatly exceeds that of the treatment itself.

In democratic countries, actual implementation of government policies by ministries and agencies reflects the true attitude toward the issue under their responsibility. In Israel, the NII is responsible for implementing governmental policy regarding victims of hostile acts. The documents show an ambivalent, hesitant policy, as well as ineffective implementation. It is true that the whole of NII work is criticized as inefficient and unwelcoming (Mizrahi et al. 2009), but the way in which it treats victims of hostilities, as a group, was explicitly criticized in the 2003 State Comptroller's Report, which called particular attention to the difficulty of navigating the eligibility-guideline maze, and stressed the need to shorten the claim-processing period.[16]

Discourse and Reality: Civil Society Organizations[17]

The vacuum left by the state-governed institutions in Israel with regard to caring for ASR and PTSD casualties has been filled by civil society organizations. These organizations were active in the field even before PTSD was publicly recognized, and provided ad hoc solutions to the mental health concerns of numerous groups. ERAN (Hebrew acronym for mental health first aid) was founded in 1971 to provide emotional first aid by telephone to people in various kinds of emotional distress. Other organizations that targeted specific populations soon followed: Professor Lahad founded the Community Stress Prevention Center (CSPC) in 1981, to address the problems encountered by residents of frontline Kiryat Shmona and other localities near the northern border. The Center for Preparedness and Coping with Emergency and Trauma (MAHUT) was established in 1988 in a similar vein, to aid residents of northern Samaria during the First Intifada (1987). Selah–Israel Crisis Management Center helps new immigrants cope with various kinds of trauma and emotional distress (established in 1993). And there are many others.

These organizations belong to the Israeli NGO sector, which has grown at an exceptional pace since the 1980s. Civil society organizations sometimes function as self-help organizations, while at other times they are frameworks that provide services that are lacking or inadequately supplied by the state, engage in advocacy, raise awareness of a myriad of issues, and seek to influence public discourse and governmental policy.[18]

Civil society organizations play a particularly crucial role in the care of trauma sufferers, whether soldiers or civilians, and their contribution to the shift from denial to recognition cannot be overstated. One such organization is Erim Balayla (Hebrew for "awake at night"), founded by a group of former POWs. Erim Balayla launched a campaign in 1997 to persuade the Defense Ministry's Rehabilitation Division to invite former POWs for assessment so that they could be accorded recognition and receive assistance and treatment.[19] The former POWs, having felt neglected by the state for years, decided to help themselves; they succeeded in making the security establishment aware of the injustice they had suffered and of the untreated post-traumatic stress disorder with which most of them were afflicted.[20] In a similar spirit of self-help, CSR casualties and military psychiatry professionals founded the Association to Advance Combat Stress Reaction Casualties in 2005. The Association's goal is to raise awareness and promote legislation that benefits CSR casualties; it is active in areas related to sufferer rights and the treatment methods practiced by the Defense Ministry's Rehabilitation Division.[21] This mode of activism also exists in other countries: it may be seen in, for example, the actions of American veteran organizations in the post–Vietnam War period, which established centers to assist trauma sufferers and pressured Congress and the professional community to advance recognition of CSR and PTSD (Blank 1985).

The leading Israeli organization in this sphere is NATAL, Israel's Trauma Center for Victims of Terror and War, which operates on behalf of soldiers and civilians who have been psychologically traumatized by events related to the Israeli-Palestinian conflict. The organization was founded in 1998 by Judith Yovel Recanati and the late Dr. Yossi Hadar. It was Hadar, then-director of Bar-Ilan University's Program in Psychotherapy, who suggested the idea for the organization. Yovel Recanati devoted herself to its execution, and has headed NATAL and guided its operations since its establishment.[22] NATAL pursues a dual goal of advocacy and service delivery. At the heart of its vision, however, is the desire to raise public awareness of the unique nature of trauma resulting from the Israeli-Palestinian conflict, and to ensure that a distinction is maintained between the sufferers of this form of trauma and those traumatized by other events, such as traffic accidents, natural disasters, or abuse. In accordance with this vision, NATAL does not confine itself to directly assisting trauma sufferers or engaging in direct advocacy vis-à-vis the governmental/security establishment. Rather, it aspires to serve as a center for advancing knowledge and awareness among the general public, not only of the suffering endured by those afflicted with trauma but also of war trauma's broader social impact. This orientation, which is specific to NATAL, dictates that the organization pursue high-profile activities that reach the widest possible audience.

NATAL's combined service/advocacy approach effectively demonstrates the advantages and disadvantages of having civil society organizations fill a vacuum left by the state. Although organizations that pursue this line of activity strive for long-term solutions (advocacy aimed at influencing public policy), they are pushed to offer immediate, if partial, assistance to their target populations. Unless the government changes its policy, the immediate, short-term assistance these organizations with limited resources can offer—important as it is—will be all there is, because governments are less inclined to invest in long-term solutions to issues allegedly taken care of by civil society. Because of its limited resources, civil society's main task should therefore be to transform governmental and public attitudes toward the issue and to promote policy changes so that the state will assume responsibility. Direct aid services are an important contribution to the welfare of the injured, but no nongovernmental, donor-funded organization can provide comprehensive, nationwide aid. When trauma casualties, like any other distressed population, are dependent on NGOs, the help they can get is limited. These organizations cannot offer psychiatric treatment to all war trauma sufferers nationwide, and they certainly are unable to fund disability benefits to those eligible. Moreover, their dependence on philanthropy frequently demands that these organizations align their work with their donors' particular preferences, which limits the scope of their actions and prevents coordination between the various organizations to distribute the aid most effectively.

The well-being of trauma casualties should not rest on the good will of a small number of generous philanthropists who might shift or cancel their support for a variety of idiosyncratic reasons. Civil society cannot ultimately replace the state. There are many reasons for government lack of resources for different social issues. In the case of war trauma, inadequacy of the government's response is due primarily to the marginalization of the issue and to the insufficient awareness that war trauma is an inevitable toll exacted by wars and hostile acts.

These limitations, which apply to all civilian organizations, are particularly highlighted by the history of the Israel Trauma Coalition (ITC), which was founded at the initiative of the UJA-Federation of New York to address the large number of sufferers of trauma caused by the Al-Aqsa Intifada.[23] The Coalition's primary mission is to coordinate fundraising and aid efforts. Its participants have included organizations that ordinarily deal with trauma and emotional distress of various kinds but that, under the exceptional circumstances of the Intifada, diverted most of their efforts toward assisting acute stress sufferers. Keren Friedman-Peleg's (2008) doctoral dissertation illustrates how dependence on funding bodies, in this case the UJA-Federation of New York, led the Coalition to make decisions that were inconsistent with the professional opinion of many of its members, and compromise on the services that it provides. She quotes several representatives of Coalition member organizations relating that heavy pressure by the donors led to increased Coalition involvement in therapist training and psycho-educational group activities aimed at building resilience and to reduce involvement in direct aid. This change in orientation was made despite the objections of many Coalition professionals who were concerned by the potential damage caused by a drastic reduction in urgently needed direct psychiatric care and assistance. A similar change of direction took place after the Second Lebanon war, when several donors limited their funding to projects focused solely on northern Israel, contrary to the position of Coalition member organizations, which felt that the termination of projects in other parts of the country, including Sderot, would cause substantial harm to the people living there. The UJA-Federation of New York also limited its financial commitment to three years, after which (in December 2005) changing priorities led to the significant decline in resources allocated to the Coalition (ibid.). Similar limitations characterize all civil society organizations, and by no means diminish the importance or value of the organizations' activity; they simply emphasize how urgent it is that the state take responsibility for these kinds of services. The advocacy practiced by civil society organizations is directed not merely toward policymakers but also toward the public at large. The immediate reason for this is obvious. Socioeconomic theory on the relationship between governmental policy and the growth of nonprofit organizations in democratic countries holds that governments tend to supply services only if they enjoy the support of the average voter. Elected officials' need for public legitimacy causes the exclusion from government funding of many services of an essentially public nature, particularly where such services target groups that lack political power.[24] Trauma sufferers fall into this category. They constitute a relatively small percentage of the electorate, and they have no political clout. By influencing public opinion and gaining support of influential figures, civil society organizations, including self-help organizations such as Erim Balayla, provide them with some political power.

Another, though less obvious, reason why civil society organizations' advocacy actions target the general public is social support. The considerable protective role of social support for casualties of CSR was discussed at length in Part I. Its importance is just as great with regard to civilians traumatized by war or catastrophe. A global meta-analysis by Fran Norris et al. (2002 [1, 2]) covering data on 60,000 disaster survivors from a large number of studies found that social support was critical to the survivors' mental health, both as a protective factor and as a coping facilitator. After the 2006 Second Lebanon War, Lahad et al. (2010), using Israeli data from that war, provided support for the foregoing findings. The authors suggest that social support exists when "the individual believes that he is being cared for and that help and assistance are available to him" (Lahad et al. 2010, p. 135; Norris et al. 2002 [1, 2]). Due to the shortage of governmental aid services, and the bureaucratic obstacles and barriers that such services pose, NGOs are filling the neglected social-support function. Their mission is to help and to prevent individuals from feeling forsaken. With the NGO in place, the individual has somewhere to turn to: someone who is concerned for her and her fate, is aware of his pain, and extends a helping hand.

The role played by the NGOs assumes yet another meaning in light of psychiatrist and Holocaust survivor Haim Dasberg's insight (noted in Part I) regarding the negative interactions that often emerge between victims of organized violence and their families/communities, and the suffering caused by these interactions. According to Dasberg, the pathological symptoms displayed by victims of organized violence elicit a rejection/labeling response, which he refers to as "complementary pathology" (Dasberg 1987, p. 101). Because the raison d'être of civil society's aid organizations is to create a warm, supportive environment and to engage the injured individual in positive interactions, their activity may be seen as therapeutic.

The therapeutic aspect or the social support of NGOs' activity is reflected, for example, in NATAL's broadcasts in the media and on its website. The broadcasts are intended both for trauma sufferers and for the general public, and they express solidarity, encouragement, and empathy for trauma sufferers. They emphasize the availability of help for the traumatized and invite them to seek assistance; at the same time, they try to evoke other viewers' sympathy and responsibility for the traumatized. To paraphrase the name of NATAL's magazine, a million copies of which are distributed annually on Israel Memorial Day, *BeNoge'a LaRegesh* (*About Feelings*; literally, touching feelings), one can say that these broadcasts aim to "touch" the emotions of the viewer.[25]

The impact of these messages is exemplified by the account of one of NATAL's first clients, an IDF reservist who had suffered post-traumatic symptoms since the First Lebanon War, and finally sought assistance after years of reserve duty that had continually reawakened his trauma.[26] He turned to NATAL during an interim period, when the IDF already had an organized professional system in place to address combat reactions, but before the phenomenon had gained sufficient societal recognition. During this period, soldiers still balked at seeking care due to fears of being stigmatized. NATAL's hassle-free, open-door policy, which is typical of all civil society organizations, made it possible for this reservist to find the courage to seek help.

The impact of NATAL and other NGOs on Israeli public discourse is difficult to measure, and even more difficult to isolate from other factors. One cannot, however, ignore the degree to which civil society activism has coincided with legislative milestones and with the growing legitimization of war trauma. The NII's new administrative order recognizing PTSD for disability rating purposes (October 2000) and the enactment of MK Zahava Galon's private bill to establish a legislative distinction between CSR and mental illness (December 2000) came three years after Erim Balayla's successful effort to change Defense Ministry policy regarding former POWs, and two years after NATAL began its public activity. NATAL successfully persuaded the NII to add a guidebook for acute stress sufferers to the National Insurance Institute website. Despite problems with the guidebook's online presentation, its inclusion confirms that the governmental/security establishment accepted NATAL's definitions and interpretations regarding the concept of war trauma.

Senior officials in the Ministry of Defense and the IDF admit that their attitudes and positions are influenced by the public activity of civil society organizations as a whole. They are, of course, also influenced by global developments in awareness and professional knowledge. The intensified professional discourse and the phenomenon's inclusion in the DSM have affected professional processes in Israel, and have thereby also influenced decision making within the government and defense establishment. There can, however, be no doubt that the issue's presence on the public agenda created a more favorable atmosphere for laws and administrative orders such as those enacted in 2000, and for overall progress with regard to trauma sufferers.

Notes

1. Also known as the Second Intifada (28 September 2000–8 February 2005).
2. On this topic, see this chapter's section "Discourse and Reality: The Governmental Establishment."
3. This is the official count: www.cbsnews.com/stories/2004/06/05/national/main 623139.shtml.
4. See Part III, Chapter 12, this volume.
5. On the dispute generated by the indirect-exposure criterion, see Rimmerman et al. (2007, p. 59). The 1994 definition was retrieved 25 June 2010 from: www.mental-health-today.com/ptsd/index.html. The foregoing description refers to Criterion A of the PTSD definition, which deals with the event. In 2000 a text revision of the DSM-IV was published, but this definition remained unchanged, meaning that it was reapproved. See DSM-IV-TR 2000.
6. Expression of Judith Lewis Herman; see Herman (1994, p. 19). This topic was addressed at length in Part I.
7. Amendment No. 8 to the Compensation for Victims of Hostile Acts Law, 20 June 1988, which expanded the criteria for recognizing disability to include "loss of the ability to perform an everyday act, whether physically or mentally, or a diminishment of that ability" (quoted in Yanay et al. 2005), p. 35.
8. Interview conducted by Zameret Hershko (a research assistant who worked with me) with Osnat Cohen, head of the NII's Victims of Hostilities Division, March 2009.
9. Statement of Ministry of Social Affairs Director-General Nahum Itzkovitz, Ninth Herzliya Conference, 2 February 2009. Retrieved 26 October 2010 from: www.her zliyaconference.org/_Uploads/2944nahomitzkovith.ppt. [Hebrew]
10. NATAL, Confidential Testimonies, Testimony NT/KA, January 2006.
11. Events that were recognizes by the state as hostile acts.

12. A southern town close to the Israeli border with the Gaza Strip, which has been suffering thousands of rocket attacks for more than 14 years.
13. "A Prosthesis for the Soul Has Yet to Be Invented" (no author specified). *HaTikva*, Terror Victims Association. Retrieved 5 July 2010 from: www.irgun.org.il. [Hebrew]
14. "Guide for Acute Stress Sufferers" (www.btl.gov.il/benefits/Victims_of_Hostilities/Pages/%D7%98%D7%99%D7%A4%D7%95%D7%9C%20%D7%A4%D7%A1%D7%99%D7%9B%D7%95%D7%9C%D7%95%D7%92%D7%99.aspx).
15. Confidential testimonies to the author, IK/YO, July 2014; IK/MM, November 2012.
16. Annual Report 54A, 2003/Payments to Victims of Hostile Acts, pp. 253–256. Retrieved 27 June 2010 from: www.mevaker.gov.il. [Hebrew]
17. This term refers to NGO organizations that constitute civil society's organized arm. For a conceptual discussion of both terms and of the broader term "civil society," see Gidron et al. (2004).
18. On the vital role played by civil society in a democracy, see Yishai (2003).
19. Interview with Miri Shalit, February 2009. See also Chapter 1, this volume.
20. The association currently numbers 300 former POWs, and engages in mutual aid, support group management, representation vis-à-vis the Defense Ministry, and the development of innovative treatment methods. Erim Balayla website: www.erim-pow.co.il/content.php?id-1, retrieved 5 April 2010.
21. Goren Committee deliberations, statement of Chaim Knobler; Ministry of Justice website, alphabetical list of associations: www.justice.gov.il/MOJHeb/NetzivutNEW/Irgunim/MugbalutNoirologit.htm, retrieved 5 April 2010. (Hebrew)
22. See NATAL website: www.natal.org.il/?CategoryID=162.
23. An in-depth discussion of the Israel Trauma Coalition and NATAL can be found in Friedman-Peleg (2008).
24. B. A. Weisbrod, cited in Gidron et al. (2004).
25. The journal and an explanation of its goals can be found on the NATAL website: www.natal.org.il/?CategoryID=162.
26. Interview with Judith Yovel Recanati, 30 July 2008.

References

American Psychiatric Association 2013, *Diagnostic and Statistical Manual of Mental Disorders*, 5th edn. Available from www.dsm5.org.

Baer, S. 2007, *Recipients of Hostile Acts Benefits, 2006*, National Insurance Institute, Research and Planning Administration. Available from www.btl.gov.il/Publications/survey%5CPages/Seker212.aspx.

Blank, A. S. 1985, 'The Veterans Administration's Viet Nam Veterans Outreach and Counseling Centers' in *The Trauma of War: Stress and Recovery in Viet Nam Veterans*, eds. S. M. Sonnenberg & A. S. Blank, American Psychiatric Press, Washington, D.C., pp. 229–238.

Bleich, A., Gelkopf, M., & Solomon, Z. 2003, 'Exposure to Terrorism, Stress-Related Mental Health Symptoms, and Coping Behaviors among a Nationally Representative Sample in Israel', *JAMA*, vol. 290, pp. 612–620.

Dasberg, H. 1987, 'Israeli Society vis-à-vis Organized Trauma, or the Therapist vis-à-vis the Survivor' in *Sichot*, vol. 1, no. 2, pp. 98–103. (Hebrew)

Friedman-Peleg, K. 2008, *The Nation on the Couch: the Use of Therapeutic Conceptualizations of Trauma and 'Resilience' in the Wake of the Al-Aqsa Intifada, the Disengagement and the Second Lebanon War*, doctoral dissertation, Tel Aviv University.

Galea, S., Ahern, J., Resnick, H., Kilpatrick, D., Bucuvalas, M., Gold, J., & Vlahov, D. 2002, 'Psychological Sequelae of the September 11 Terrorist Attacks in New York City', *New England Journal of Medicine*, vol. 346, no. 13, pp. 982–987.

Gidron, B., Bar, M., & Katz, H. 2004, *The Israeli Third Sector: between Welfare State and Civil Society*, Kluwer Academic/Plenum, New York.

Herman, J. L. 1994, *Trauma and Recovery*, Basic Books, New York.

Kessler, R. C. 2000, 'Post-Traumatic Stress Disorder: the Burden to the Individual and to Society', *Journal of Clinical Psychiatry*, vol. 61, no. 5, pp. 4–12.

Lahad, M., Shacham, M., & Shacham, Y. 2010, 'The Impact of the Second Lebanon War on the Experience of Trauma and on the Resilience of Jews and Arabs in Northern Israel: a Longitudinal Study', in *Health, Education and Welfare Services in Times of Crisis: Lessons Learned from the Second Lebanon War*, eds. F. Azaiza, N. Nachmias, & M. Cohen, Pardes, Haifa, pp. 117–144. (Hebrew)

Levy, A., Witztum, E., Granek, M., & Kotler, M. 1990, 'The Treatment of Combat Stress Reaction in the IDF, 1948–1973', *Harefuah*, vol. 32, pp. 49–53.

Mizrahi, S., Vigoda-Gadot, E., & Cohen, N. 2009, 'Trust, Participation and Performance', *Public Management Review*. Available from http://poli.haifa.ac.il/~eranv/material_vigoda/PMR.pdf [26 June 2010].

Neria, Y., Gross, R., & Marshall R. D. 2006, 'Mental Health in the Wake of Terrorism: Making Sense of Mass Casualty Trauma', in *9/11: Mental Health in the Wake of Terrorist Attacks*, eds. Y. Neria, R. Gross, & R. D. Marshall, Cambridge University Press, New York.

Norris, F. H., Friedman, M. J., & Watson, P. J. 2002, 1, '60,000 Disaster Victims Speak: Part II. Summary and Implications of the Disaster Mental Health Research', *Psychiatry*, vol. 65, pp. 240–260.

Norris, F. H., Friedman, M. J., Watson, P. J., Byrne, C. M., Diaz, E., & Kaniasty, K. 2002, 2, '60,000 Disaster Victims Speak: Part I. An Empirical Review of the Empirical Literature, 1981–2001', *Psychiatry*, vol. 65, pp. 207–239.

Regulant-Levy, R. 1994, *The Thesis of Personal Recovery: the Coping Patterns of PTSD-Afflicted Civilians Undergoing Psychotherapy*, master's degree thesis, School of Social Work, Hebrew University. (Hebrew)

Rimmerman, A., Tal-Katz, P., & Avrami, S. 2007, 'People Injured in Acts of Terror in Israel and the United states: a Comparative Review and Future Recommendations', *Social Security*, vol. 73, pp. 41–68. (Hebrew)

Schuster, M. A., Stein, B. D., Jaycox, L. H., Collins, R. L., Marshall, G. N., Elliott, M. N., Zhou, A. J., Kanouse, D. E., Morrison, J. L., & Berry, S. H. 2001, 'A National Survey of Stress Reactions after the September 11, 2001 Terrorist Attacks', *New England Journal of Medicine*, vol. 345, pp. 1507–1512.

Somer, E., & Bleich, A. 2005, 'Stress in a Population under Prolonged Terrorist Attack: Identification, Characterization and Treatment Challenges' in *Mental Health in Terror's Shadow: the Israeli Experience*, eds. E. Somer & A. Bleich, Ramot, Tel Aviv, pp. 9–26. (Hebrew)

Yanay, U., Prior, R., & Baer, S. 2005, *Victims of Hostile Acts in Israel: Injuries, Needs, Legislation and the Delivery of Services and Assistance*, School of Social Work, Hebrew University and the Research and Planning Authority, the National Insurance Institute, Jerusalem. (Hebrew)

Yishai, Y. 2003, *Civil Society in Israel*, Carmel, Haifa. (Hebrew)

10 The Trauma Discourse Dialectic

Trauma discourse, all over the world, has always been intertwined with views, images, and ethos of heroism. The traumatic syndrome, which has been confused with weakness of character, has frightened and misled generals, physicians, and psychiatrists, who erroneously contrasted it with heroism. This misperception, together with the persistent power of prejudice and suspicion, created what is now recognized as a "historical professional error," which caused war trauma casualties enormous, extended suffering (Levy et al. 1990; Bleich 2000; Chapter 1, this volume).

Heroism discourse everywhere also affects other sensitive painful issues related to casualties of war, such as medals and honors awarded to soldiers according to the nature and location of their actions, and their war-related injuries or death. Such awards evoke bitter, upsetting disputes concerning eligibility, which reflect an aching yearning of the casualties and their families to be embraced by the nation on behalf of whom they lost so much, especially because heroism is glorified by society. Such desires, however, encounter determined efforts to limit the number of awards, to ensure that the honor remains—they believe—unique and admired.

The heroism discourse makes it so much harder to accept that trauma is no less a legitimate injury than a physical one. When discussing civilians, this clash of images interlaces with the fact that they are usually not the protectors but the protected. They send the soldiers to defend them at war, and glorify their sacrifice and heroism.

For this reason, this chapter opens with a discussion of the efforts of Israeli civilians to gain recognition as equal contributors to the county's existential struggle—and to be considered heroes, just like soldiers. The Israeli case is more intense than the case of other Western countries, as war and terror have affected both soldiers and civilians throughout Israel's entire years of existence. It still, however, sheds light on similar issues in other countries, such as the issue of how to decorate and how to remember the civilian victims of 9/11, or of the July 2005 London bombing. Most victims of terror attacks are civilians, who are targeted by terrorism in the midst of their daily life. Some, including civilians, are injured or killed while helping to save others. These issues of recognition and honor apply to them all.

Civilians, Soldiers, and the Israeli Heroism Scale

Efforts to raise the status of civilians on the Israeli heroism scale (see Chapter 7, this volume) began in the 1970s, but escalated to a bitter public dispute in full force two decades later, in the second half of the 1990s. The large number of fatalities and injuries sustained on the home front during the period following the Oslo Accords[1] spurred the victims of hostile acts and their families to fight for official state recognition of their contribution to Israel's existential struggle. As a result of the altered character of warfare that emerged during the Gulf War, and the spread of armed conflict in the form of terrorist attacks on Israel's major cities, Israeli civilians once again identified with Ben-Gurion's statement during the War of Independence: "The entire people is the army, the entire land is the warfront."[2] Ironically, this statement that was originally meant to raise civilian morale and enlist civilians' support in Israel's war for independence was never followed through to its logical conclusion: if all the entire population is the army, then it is justified (actually, natural) to memorialize civilian victims of hostile acts the same way as the fallen soldiers. Although most of the material rights of civilian victims were equalized to those of soldiers in 1970, government policy consistently perpetuated a separation of the two groups, justified by ideological arguments emphasizing solders' special role in the nation's defense.[3]

The campaign waged by the victims of hostile acts, while directed mainly toward symbolic recognition of their contribution, also sought to create an official framework of social support for more than 20,000 injured, 1,700 killed civilians, and their families[4] in Israel, corresponding to that established by wounded-veteran organizations and by organizations for bereaved military families. This administrative aspect of the campaign scored a victory in 1997, when the Terror Victims Association (TVA), headed at the time by Dov Kalmanovich, who had himself been critically wounded in a terrorist attack in 1988, was recognized as a "representative organization." This status, as defined by law, conferred upon the organization the right to represent its members vis-à-vis the state institutions that deliberated over applications for both material rights and symbolic privileges. Nonetheless, despite the formal equalization of the rights of victims of hostilities with those of wounded Israel Defense Forces (IDF) soldiers, many differences between the rights of victims of hostilities and those of wounded IDF soldiers remained. According to the TVA's current chairperson (since 2011), Tzvika Shahak, these differences constitute discrimination against the civilian wounded. For example, there is no national support system to help victims and their families during the first hours and days after an incident, as exists for IDF soldiers; the TVA receives no funding for its activities on behalf of orphans and widows, making it hard for the organization to engage in the kind of welfare activity conducted by the Defense Ministry vis-à-vis bereaved IDF families.[5] Moreover, terrorist attacks on the home front often injure more than one family member, sometimes both parents, and in certain cases, entire families. In such circumstances, a single family might have experienced both deaths and injuries, making for a multilayered situation, encompassing bereavement, physical disability, psychological trauma, and, often, the loss of the family's source of emotional and financial support. No satisfactory solution has yet been found for such complexity of distress, as indicated by, for example, the lack of an official definition of the status of orphans who lost both of their parents in hostile acts.[6]

Despite the foregoing differences in the treatment of civilian and military victims, a 2003 survey conducted by the TVA shows that the majority of wounded civilians felt that their material needs were adequately met. Most of the survey respondents stated that the obstacles they were facing in the material sphere were not very different from those faced by those wounded during military service. In their opinion, both groups have trouble getting information and answers within the bureaucratic maze; both feel powerless vis-à-vis the medical committees (in charge of determining eligibility and extent of indemnification); some of the needs of both groups go unmet; and both groups encounter obstacles of various kinds while seeking to obtain services and to exercise their rights (Even 2007).

The heart of the struggle waged by the victims of hostile acts appears to be over the symbolic aspects of recognition and commemoration, the absence of which creates a situation that Shahak describes as one of great loneliness for the victims. "Like being the less-loved child," he says, "as the nation and the community mainly embrace and honor soldiers and show families of wounded civilians less affection."[7] Shahak's personal experience unwittingly places him at the center of Israel's heroism-scale dilemma: he has been on both sides of the soldier-civilian divide. As a young Navy lieutenant and commander of the Daburim unit[8] in the Yom Kippur war (1973), he was awarded the Medal for Distinguished Service for extricating soldiers under fire in the Gulf of Suez. In that war, his wife Ayelet's uncle was killed in the Golan Heights. Twenty-three years later, in March 1996, Tzvika and Ayelet lost their eldest daughter, 15-year-old Bat-Chen, in a terrorist attack by a suicide bomber at Tel Aviv's Dizengoff Shopping Center. Possibly, owing to this tragic combination of losses, Shahak is well entitled to suggest that the struggle for recognition does not aim to achieve absolute parity between soldiers and civilians, but rather to have them recognized one alongside the other. This is exemplified in the request to designate space at the Mount Herzl national cemetery and memorial facility for all of Israel's fallen sons and daughters. In his words, "I don't compare my daughter who was murdered at Dizengoff Center to my wife's uncle who was killed on Yom Kippur defending Israel on the Golan Heights. They don't have to occupy the same place on the heroism scale, but both of them do have a place on it."[9]

The victims of hostile acts do not dispute the Israeli heroism ethos, but rather wish to become incorporated within it as full and equal partners. This desire is rooted in a profound need to confer meaning on the loss of one's loved ones and on the suffering of those still alive—the injured and their families. A sense of meaning can help the bereaved recover and the wounded cope with their injuries. Both groups, civilians and soldiers, cling firmly to such meaning, which is reflected in official and social recognition of the enormity of their unique sacrifice, and both groups have become embroiled in a bitter and painful struggle that has been raging in Israel for the past 15 years. Bereaved IDF families view equivalent commemoration as depreciation of official state recognition accorded to soldiers, inasmuch as it disregards the difference in intent between the military and civilian casualties: "How can you compare our fallen with those killed in a café?" remonstrated Pnina Cohen, then-chair of the IDF Widows and Orphans Organization, in May 2000 (Lapid 2000). Her attitude was not uncommon. The year of the government decision to hold a state memorial ceremony for civilians killed in hostile acts (1998) was also a year characterized by a broad public consensus on the supremacy of military bereavement on the social-status scale (Kim 1998). This consensus stems from the concept that although civilians pay with their lives for belonging to the nation, their presence at the site of a given terrorist incident is random—whether they are at work or at play—and their deaths serve only to underscore the importance of the army, which protects the home front from even greater dangers. "You can't compare someone who fought [in combat] with someone who was walking down the street when an evil terrorist planted a bomb that caused his death," says Asa Kasher (a leading philosopher in Israel, who is credited with writing the IDF Code of Ethics), who lost his son Yehoraz while serving as an IDF officer in 1991. "[The person walking down the street] didn't volunteer to risk his life, he didn't volunteer to serve, he wasn't devoting all of his time and energy and thoughts to defending the state and its citizens."[10]

For their part, the families of those injured in hostile acts felt that the second-rate recognition accorded to their sacrifice, such as an absence of official commemorative activities for wounded civilians, was tantamount to having their loved ones' names erased from the nation's collective memory. The depth of the emotions evoked by this debate is reflected in a statement by Smadar Haran-Kaiser, who lost her husband and both of her daughters in a terrorist attack in Nahariya in 1979. Haran-Kaiser views the secondary status accorded to civilian terrorism victims as the final phase in the enemy's designs to "wipe us off the face of the earth." She argues that maintaining one's everyday routine despite the constant danger on buses, in markets, and along the borders is a form of heroism no less estimable than that of soldiers going out to battle (Haran-Kaiser, quoted in Lapid, 2000). Her words echo Moshe Dayan's 1956 eulogy for Ro'i Rotenberg, in which he glorified civilians' continual willingness to pursue all of their normal activities, in all parts of the country, despite the danger.[11] Forty years later, the families of wounded civilians requested the recognition of such civilian heroism as fully comparable to the heroism of Israel's military fallen, and as due an equal place in the nation's symbols and ceremonies. Since the terrorist attacks of the 1990s, and even more strongly since the Al-Aqsa Intifada (2000–2004), the families of victims of hostile acts have demanded full equality, including complete unification of memorial ceremonies and an end to all bereavement hierarchies. They argue that in the "home front war," as they have referred to the events of the 2000s, shopping malls, cafés, buses, pubs, and restaurants have all become combat areas, making a "distinction between the two types of bereavement [. . .] archaic, unrealistic, and immoral" (Karman et al. 2004).

Under pressure from victims and their families, in 1998 the Netanyahu government decided to supplement official events on Israel's Memorial Day for fallen IDF soldiers with a ceremony honoring those killed in hostile acts, and a monument was erected for them as well. The ceremony, however, was to be held two hours after the ceremony for soldiers. In both groups, the decision attracted supporters and opponents. The victims of hostile acts were not content with a supplementary ceremony and wished to be included in the events honoring fallen IDF soldiers. Their representative Tzvika Shahak takes a more moderate line. He does not seek a joint ceremony that blurs the distinctions between soldiers and civilians, but proposes a single ceremony composed of two parts, enabling equal but separate attention to both groups.[12] The debate has not been resolved, and there are many places in Israel where no ceremony at all is held for the victims of hostile acts, due to the objections of Yad Labanim, an influential organization that commemorates fallen soldiers and assists bereaved IDF families. On the other hand, the parents of fallen soldiers found the decision to erect a monument to civilian casualties to be offensive. They felt that such a monument violates the unspoken rule that Mount Herzl house only monuments honoring those who fell while serving in Israel's security forces or soldiers who have no graves or whose burial sites are difficult to visit. Professor Avraham (Rami) Friedman, who lost his soldier son David in 1984, argues that not only does equal official commemoration devaluate the principle of soldierly intention and sense of mission, but also the monument has created a situation in which the civilians killed in hostile acts have, as it were, two commemoration sites: a monument at Mount Herzl and a civilian grave in their local towns.[13]

Yossi Tzur, whose son Assaf was killed in a 2003 terrorist attack in Haifa, perfectly expresses the position of unifying all commemoration lineaments of the two groups. In a speech he delivered on behalf of the victims of hostile acts in April 2010 at the state memorial ceremony at Mount Herzl, Tzur demanded full equalization of all aspects of state commemoration activities, including the terminology used to describe both groups:

> After over a century of struggle for our right to live here, and after sixty-two years of independence, the ethos of military and civilian heroism is becoming unified. The Israeli heroism ethos is no longer found on battlefields far from the major cities and civilian population centers [. . .] The time has [also] come to stop using the term "victims of hostile acts" to describe those who have fallen due to acts of terrorism. The terminology that the state has chosen to employ affects the status of those killed by terrorism, it designates them as inferior, second-class fallen. A declaration that those killed in terrorist attacks are included among those who have fallen in Israel's wars would put an end to this form of discrimination.
>
> (Tzur 2010)

Distinguishing between military and civilian casualties is an accepted practice among all Western nations, and has been common since the first military cemeteries were established. In July 1862, the US Congress passed a law that laid the foundations worldwide for separate commemoration of those who fell in the service of their nation. The law states that those who sacrificed their lives defending the Republic during the Civil War should be interred in "national cemeteries [. . .] enclosed with a good and substantial stone or iron fence" (quoted in Mosse 1990, pp. 56–57). In Europe, the systematic burial of soldiers apart from civilians began toward the end of the nineteenth century, during the Franco-Prussian War (1870–1871). In World War I, the custom of burying fallen soldiers in common graves at the battle site was utterly abandoned, and military ceremonies were held in symbolic glorification of the nation's heroes (Mosse 1990). The practice of separate burial still prevails today. Even in exceptional circumstances, as in the state commemoration of the over 60,000 British civilians who died in World War II, a strict separation is upheld between the military and civilian spheres in terms of cemetery maintenance and memorialization of the deceased. UK civilians killed more recently in terrorist acts committed by the Irish Republican Army (IRA) were not accorded state commemoration. Moreover, financial compensation for the victims of IRA attacks in the UK was disassociated from any national defense context, and provided via the same compensation framework as that for victims of criminal activity (Even 2007). This distinction was also maintained with respect to the July 2005 London underground bombing: a collective memorial for the 52 civilians killed (in addition to more than 700 injured) is located in Hyde Park. This is actually the reverse of what has happened in Israel: the UK went from full state recognition of the civilian role in World War II to a categorical distinction between soldiers and those killed in hostile acts, while in Israel the struggle to erase this separation is still underway.

The September 11, 2001, terror attack on the US raised the issue of civilian commemoration in the US. Despite the sense of war in the home front caused by this catastrophic attack, the US government maintained its traditional distinction between soldiers and civilians. Two weeks after the attack, the American Department of Defense created the "Defense of Freedom Medal," which was awarded to 90 nonuniformed workers who were supporting the Defense Department and killed or injured in the attack, designated as "defense civilians." The medal was declared the civilian equivalent to the military Purple Heart (Cahlink 2001). Ten years, however, were needed for the Congress and Senate to approve a bill commissioning the US Treasury to design and strike three Congressional Gold Medals to honor the nearly 3,000 civilians killed that day, who were not considered defense civilians (Rein 2011).

One of the ideas that the families of victims of hostile acts find hardest to bear is that their loved ones were randomly targeted by a terrorist attack that caught them in the midst of what should have been an ordinary day. This random-death belief erases all meaning from the bereaved families' anguish and makes it all the harder for them to deal with their loss. In their eyes, the intentionality criteria does not justify what they regard as the exclusion of civilian casualties from the heroism scale, because—for them—the very fact that someone was killed in downtown Tel Aviv makes him or her "part of Israel's war."[14]

The problem with satisfying the civilian need for recognition is that similar concerns of depleted meaning are precisely what drive the families of fallen soldiers to oppose equal status for "those killed in cafés" and soldiers killed while defending the nation. Recognition of one's unique, intentional contribution to the homeland plays a crucial role in motivating soldiers to consciously risk their lives, and in ensuring the willingness of all citizens to continue to send their children to combat service. The symbolic framework of honor encourages soldiers and their families to continue shouldering the burden of sacrifice for the sake of the collective. The comparison to a civilian injured in the course of his everyday activities threatens the validity of this recognition. Given the reality of Israeli life, in which an impending sense of catastrophe coexists with the duty to risk one's life for the sake of the nation, an emphasis on intention and sense of mission confer national-existential meaning on a soldier's willingness to fight, as do the continued expressions of public gratitude (Witztum & Malkinson 1993).

The debate over official recognition of the sacrifice made by civilian casualties is closely connected to the denial/recognition process of psychological trauma as a legitimate injury, and can explain why the campaign to equalize the status of civilian casualties on the home front to that of soldiers borrows its vocabulary from the Israeli mythology of strength and heroism. Psychological trauma is regarded in Israel as a sign of weakness in spite of its formal legitimacy, and is even thought to undermine the fortitude of Israeli society as a whole. Asa Kasher argues that this is one of the reasons why so few sought psychological care during the Al-Aqsa Intifada. In his view, the individual civilian feels that he should not be weaker than the collective and fears that a quest for assistance would be looked upon as compromising the overall resilience of Israeli society (Kasher 2005). Acute stress is thus thought to undermine the image of the courageous civilian, and subvert his depiction as a hero who "refuses to give in to fear" and remains steadfastly at his post, whether in the market or on the bus (Haran-Kaiser, quoted in Lapid 2000). However, the large number of acute stress sufferers also calls attention to the high price paid by civilians in wartime, and stimulates discussion of the idea of a "home front war." A dialectic has thus emerged that, while stressing the role of civilians, "corrects" the dissonance created by their equalization to soldiers, and emphasizes the fact that those injured in hostile acts are helpless victims, not combatants.

War Trauma and National Resilience

National resilience became a topic of heated public debate due to the growing number of acute stress reaction (ASR) sufferers produced by the Al-Aqsa Intifada, and to fears that there might be a grain of truth in Hassan Nasrallah's remark that Israel is weaker than a "spider's web." In practice, the resilience displayed by Israeli society during the Second Intifada contradicted this prophecy of doom, and greatly exceeded even society's own expectations.

Scholars agree that Israeli society maintained its stability during the Intifada, and that the Israeli public recovered quickly and resumed its normal routine even following periods of high-frequency terrorist attacks (Elran 2006; Gal 2003; Ben-Dor et al. 2007). For example, out-of-home excursions, which were significantly reduced in response to the Intifada, began to revert to normal levels well before its end. Movie theater visits reached a record low in 2002 when the number and intensity of terrorist attacks peaked, but gradually rose shortly afterward and returned to pre-Intifada levels in 2004 (Elran 2006). Data also indicate that the Israeli economy recovered quite quickly: economic growth, which all but vanished during the first years of the Intifada, resumed in 2003 and quickly soared to 5.2% in 2005.[15] The Israeli public also improved its capacity for emotional adjustment to the circumstances, which is evident from Israeli Center for Victims of Terror and War (NATAL) hotline usage statistics during the Intifada, where changes in hotline usage levels may be taken as indicators of change in general anxiety levels. In 2003, this call rate returned to its pre-Intifada levels, and from then onward maintained a consistently moderate level of activity with only occasional spikes in activity.[16]

Despite the evidence of rapid recovery and resumption of normal life, Israeli public discourse during the Al-Aqsa Intifada was preoccupied with the growing number of ASR diagnoses and with implications of such diagnoses for national security and resilience. In fact, the concept of national resilience in Israel at that time was almost exclusively tied to individual attitudes and behaviors concerning security issues. It was the social justice protest of summer 2011 that highlighted the socioeconomic aspects of national resilience.

The term "resilience" initially gained popularity in the psychological literature of the 1970s, where it was used to denote the individual's efforts to deal with everyday problems. Over time, the term was increasingly employed in discussions of communal fortitude in the face of crisis, and was defined as the ability to recover quickly from adversity and resume one's everyday routine—which might itself be modified to suit the new circumstances (Zigelman et al. n.d.). The first community-resilience development programs were launched in Israel in the 1980s by the education system, as preventive efforts to help teachers and school-based treatment personnel cultivate coping skills among children exposed to war, terrorism, and loss. These community-based programs were oriented toward helping small, homogeneous communities, particularly border localities and settlements in the Occupied Territories,[17] to withstand prolonged security threats (Elran 2006). During the Al-Aqasa Intifada in the early 2000s, after a few years of intensive involvement with post-trauma, clinicians have increasingly called for a new approach, such as post-traumatic growth (positive psychological change as a result of the struggle with traumatic circumstances), to be employed in addition to efforts to prevent or heal pathology (Bleich 2006, 2007). In response, new programs have been launched, aimed at developing individual and communal coping resources for times of emergency and stress.

During the Al-Aqsa period, the Israeli public realized that the national-security conflict is no longer being conducted solely between armies, but rather, and perhaps primarily, on the civilian home front. This led to concerns for the impact of a decline in public morale and the collective's ability to handle the tension and suffering of war, prompting efforts to measure the "social component of national resilience."[18] The problem with this measurement project, which employs attitude surveys and public opinion polls, is its emphasis on the individual's role in national resilience, indirectly placing on the individual almost exclusive responsibility for collective (national) resilience. Such a conception of national resilience is inconsistent with the original meaning of the term, which encompasses also societal resilience at the macro level, in a wide variety of contexts, of which security is only one. Although resilience lies at the intersection of individual response to distress and communal or societal response to ongoing crisis, national resilience is more than the sum of individual coping abilities (Amit & Fleischer 2005). The focus on war and security events deflects attention from the fact that national-societal resilience in a democratic society is a multidimensional phenomenon, one that incorporates elements of solidarity and cohesion, social, economic, and political rights; equality; and social, economic, and cultural rifts (Friedman et al. 2003; Arian et al. 2003; Friedland 2005). This means that one of its important features is mutual solidarity between the state and its citizens.

Interestingly, although the concept of national resilience remains vague, with no well-accepted theoretical conceptualization, the term has been readily embraced in Israel—notwithstanding its inadequate measurement indices—and its research is expanding in cooperation between trauma researchers and scholars of national and defense strategy.[19] Preoccupation with national resilience intensified after the Second Lebanon War (2006), which plunged Israel into chaos, exposed its lack of preparedness for rocket attacks on its civilian population, and triggered high levels of civilian anxiety. However, its current conceptualization limits its potential contribution to the development of personal and communal strategies for coping with crisis. At times, the intense preoccupation with national resilience seems like an imagined solution to Israel's as-yet unresolved ideological-emotional qualms surrounding the legitimacy and meaning of war-related acute stress reactions.

Overemphasis on the role of individual civilian resilience in national security is underscored by the parameters currently used to measure the societal component of national resilience, which were formulated during the Second Intifada. In 2003—relating to the Al-Aqsa Intifada—Israel's National Security Council proposed to define resilience as "Israeli society's ability to withstand ongoing difficulties," stressing criteria of psychological, sociological, and adjustment ability of Israeli citizens (Gal 2003). The Israeli National Security Council's definition also includes a behavioral dimension, as measured by data such as emergency hotline usage, recreational outings, and crime and violence levels. As shown earlier in this chapter, these indictors indicated high resilience of Israelis. A group of scholars from Haifa University suggested a different definition and criteria, within their newly developed index for the social component of national resilience (Haifa Indicators), which is published annually. They defined national resilience as "the ability of individuals in a given society that is involved in a protracted conflict to maintain stability with regard to the basic perceptions and beliefs which together construct their collective social fabric" (Ben-Dor et al. 2007).[20] Both definitions, however, focus on the micro level—that is, on the endurance of individuals—and include ideological dimensions, such as commitment to the state and patriotism, as well as emotional-cognitive dimensions, such as fear and optimism (Gal 2003).[21] To highlight the problematic nature of Israel's prevailing definition of national resilience, a more detailed discussion of the dimensions of commitment and patriotism follows.

The commitment to stand strong in the face of crisis is regarded in psychological literature as a key indicator of an individual's resilience. Suzanne Kobasa, a leading scholar in the field, views it as one of three main variables, along with sense of challenge and sense of control, that determine whether an individual deals successfully with the problems he faces (Mills & Dombeck 2005). Michal Shamai (2010) argues, in line with Kobasa's theory, that because war situations are forced upon civilians due to their affiliation with their state, their commitment to cope with such situations is rooted in their commitment to the state. One can look at it this way: a commitment to the state imposes upon civilians, among other things, a responsibility to maintain stability, social order, and national morale, and therefore implies an obligation to handle adequately any difficult national circumstance to which they have been subjected. Without this sense of commitment, most civilians would try to flee the country whenever war breaks out. In fact, the enemy targets civilians specifically to weaken this sense of commitment, hoping public opinion will consequently induce the leadership to change its policies (Elran 2006). Thus, civilians' ability to maintain a stable commitment to the state even under stress and crisis situations has implications for the state's ability to face its challenges. From this perspective, the patriotism and commitment-to-the-state parameters used to measure national resilience seem appropriate.

The main problems with the commitment parameter in measuring national resilience are its imbalanced focus on the individual and its failure to take into account the reciprocity between the individual and the state. Thus, argues Shamai, Israel entered the Second Lebanon War with weak and inadequate social, health, and educational services, due to a lengthy and aggressive privatization policy that directly conveyed the following message to citizens: "The state is no longer responsible for the welfare of its residents; you will have to fend for yourselves." According to Shamai, this failed reciprocity reached a peak in the summer of 2006, when the state did not provide for the required preparedness of the bombarded areas. In other words, the state did not display solidarity with its own citizens, thus threatening the sense of commitment necessary for resilience and for effectively coping with the formidable challenges of war, which occurred both in the battlefield and on the home front. Shamai's view meshes well with the definition of societal support, proposed by Lahad et al. (2010), according to which such support exists when the individual believes that he is being cared for, and that help and assistance are available to him. When the individual lacks assurance of such care, she feels alienated and alone, and her ability to face the challenges of war is diminished.

In other words, measuring citizens' commitment to the state as a component of resilience, without including in this measure the critical component of perceived state-citizen reciprocity, imposes on citizens the sole responsibility for societal-national resilience. Such an approach ignores the significance of formal social support systems in coping with traumatic situations, or rather the impact of a lack thereof. The state's diminishing role in social service provision thus has ramifications that extend beyond the difficulties faced by civilians in everyday life. Privatization of social services significantly reduces the degree of social support available to Israelis and is eroding their sense of solidarity, and consequently adversely affects Israel's national resilience. This view is consistent with the conclusions reached by Karin Amit and Nicole Fleischer, who compared Israeli and international approaches to societal resilience, and with the work of Avraham (Rami) Friedman and his colleagues on cohesion as a component of societal resilience (Amit & Fleischer 2005; Friedman et al. 2003). These studies support the argument that in order for individuals to find the inner fortitude necessary to cope with the challenges facing the collective, they must feel protected and enjoy a sense of equity in the state's distribution of resources and burdens. Ideally, they should view the state as a source of support in times of emergency or crisis. These two forms of commitment—the state's commitment to its citizens and citizens' commitment to the state—are interdependent, and individual fortitude in the face of crisis affects and is affected by the macro level of social practice.

A clear example of the relationship between impaired solidarity and poor resilience is the situation of Sderot. During the period 2001–2009, some 10,000 Kassam rockets were fired on the town.[22] Nine of its residents were killed by the rockets, along with 19 residents of neighboring localities. These numbers might seem low, but given Sderot's overall population of 19,000 (according to Central Bureau of Statistics data for 2008) it is equivalent to 2,700 deaths at a national level, or 950 if the same percentage were to die in a city with a population the size of Rhode Island. The gravity of the situation notwithstanding, during peacetime Sderot remains far from the public eye, with occasional national media coverage at best, and most of the burden of assisting its residents is being borne by civil society rather than state organizations that offer psychological and financial assistance. According to a 2007 study by NATAL, Sderot residents are afflicted with full or partial PTSD at rates higher than both the national average and rates in the Gaza Perimeter, most of them kibbutzim,[23] which faces similar risks. The researchers found a direct link between Sderot's socioeconomic status and socio-geographic marginality and the high prevalence of PTSD among its inhabitants. Moreover, within Sderot itself differences in the rate of PTSD were found between the affluent and the poor, whose coping resources were minimal and who enjoy practically no social support (Berger & Gelkopf 2007). These conclusions are consistent with other findings of the study, which indicate that Sderot residents' sense of belonging to their local community and to the state is much lower than that of the Gaza Perimeter residents. The kibbutzim are mostly inhabited by a stronger socioeconomic population, the majority of whom joined the kibbutzim by choice, while many of Sderot's inhabitants are second and third generation to immigrants who were sent there by the government in the 1950s, directly after their immigration to Israel. Based on their findings, the researchers attribute the high percentage of PTSD among Sderot's residents to their lower coping resources, which are due more to their socioeconomic marginality, their neglect by the Israeli central government, and their sense of having been forgotten and abandoned by the state than to other differences between them and the inhabitants of the neighboring localities.

When it comes to weakened populations, psychologist Rony Berger, an expert on disaster intervention who has worked for many years from a mobile NATAL unit in Sderot, maintains that states all over the world tend to fail to assume responsibility for their citizens during and in the aftermath of natural disasters, military action, and terrorist attacks (Berger 2007). According to Berger, a conspiracy of silence exists between trauma sufferers and the authorities, in which trauma sufferers' preference to refrain from seeking assistance plays into the hands of the authorities. Avoidance of reminders of their trauma, including seeking assistance, is a well-known symptom of trauma victims, along with the fear of being stigmatized and of being unable to obtain services. The authorities, on their part, whether knowingly or unknowingly, withhold assistance, particularly when those injured belong to less-affluent sectors in the geographic and socioeconomic periphery, because those citizens' voice is less heard by the public. Linking this analysis to Michal Shamai's study, one cannot but wonder about states' role in making it much harder for their citizens to obtain the very resilience that governments expect.

The aforementioned definitions and criteria of the societal component of national resilience in Israel are furthermore challenged by the relationship between coping ability, fear, and patriotism. In light of the different ways in which "patriotism" is understood by Israel's various population sectors, the very use of patriotism as a component of national resilience assessment is problematic. The inappropriateness becomes all the more obvious when we look at the items employed to measure patriotism levels in the Haifa Indicators, at least two of which encapsulate the controversial nature of the term itself. These items are average responses to these statements: "When Israel is condemned abroad, I am offended," and "When the security situation requires it, a tax increase is justified." The first statement implies that anyone willing to accept criticism of Israel in certain situations is unpatriotic, and that a patriot is a person who identifies the government with the state, and cannot acknowledge that the government's policies might be worthy of condemnation. Similarly, the tax-increase statement implies automatic support for the way in which the government distributes its resources. The main problem in incorporating patriotism as a component of resilience, however, lies in the linkage that it posits between patriotism and uncontrollable emotions, such as fear or optimism, or psychological injuries, such as trauma. If patriotism and national resilience are one and the same, as this approach would have us believe, then anyone who doubts the justice of Israel's reason in a particular war is not resilient, and anyone whose resilience falters is necessarily unpatriotic. A linkage of this type indicates that war trauma is still far from legitimation. It echoes, albeit subtly, the archaic idea that love of one's country can prevent CSR or ASR.

Notes

1. During the period of 1993–1996, Palestinian terrorists of Hamas and Jihad, who objected to the agreements, executed a series of terror attacks in the center of Israeli towns and cities. A total of 132 Israelis were killed in 11 suicide bombings, and over 100 were killed in dozens of stabbings and shootings. Hundreds were wounded. Most of the casualties were civilians.
2. "The Home Front across the Timeline," retrieved 5 February 2010 from: www.oref.org.il/82-he/PAKAR.aspx. (Hebrew)
3. See the section "The Heroism Scale during the Transition from Charity to Rights," Chapter 7, this volume.
4. See Chapter 7, this volume.
5. Conversation of the author with Tzvika Shahak, chair of the Terror Victims Organization, on 26 May 2011 (henceforth "Shahak interview, 2011").
6. Shahak interview, 2011.
7. Shahak interview, 2011.
8. An Israeli Navy unit of patrol boats.
9. Shahak interview, 2011.
10. Interview for Nurit Kedar's film *The Bereavement Wars* (quoted in Klein 2006).
11. See Chapter 7, this volume.
12. Shahak interview, 2011.
13. Author's interview with Prof. Rami Friedman, 12 July 2010.
14. Shahak interview, 2011.
15. Letter of the governor of the Bank of Israel, Stanley Fischer, to the Government and the Knesset Finance Committee, 2 April 2006. Retrieved 29 January 2010 from: www.bankisrael.gov.il/en/NewsAndPublications/RegularPublications/Pages/Doch2005/Nagid2005.aspx.
16. The NATAL hotline usage data were obtained by the author from the organization in March 2009. One should interpret these data with caution. Help-seeking behavior indicates confidence in the availability of social support, which can itself facilitate coping with stress. Furthermore, the ability to acknowledge one's difficulties and to seek coping strategies may actually attest to considerable resilience. By contrast, a failure to seek help may indicate fears of negative labeling and of being declared a burden on society.
17. The Occupied Territories refer to the territories conquered by Israel in 1967, in the West Bank (also known as Judea and Samaria) and before 2005 also the Gaza Strip, from which Israel withdrew on that year.
18. The term was included in the Haifa Indices, 2003.
19. See the relevant cooperative effort between the Reut Institute and the Israel Trauma Coalition: Reut Institute, 2009, "Reshet Hossen Ezrahit" (concept for national and local security in Israel [Hebrew]), retrieved September 2011 from http://reutinstitute.org/Data/Uploads/Articles%20and%20Reports%20from%20other%20organizations/20091026%20-%20Civil%20Resilience%20Network%20-%20PDF%20Hebrew%20-%20Version%20B%20FV.pdf.
20. The National Security Studies Center at the University of Haifa has been addressing these issues in the framework of its "Haifa Indicators" since the beginning of the Al-Aqsa Intifada, based on this definition of national resilience.
21. See Ben-Dor (2003). On definitions of resilience in its personal and adjustment-oriented sense, see Bleich (2006, 2007).
22. According to the Sderot—Tikshoret Hevratit (social media) website, "What You Need to Know about Qassams", retrieved 9 August 2009 from: http://sderotmedia.org.il/bin/content.cgi?ID=388&q=6&s=16.
23. Kibbutzim are small collective communities in Israel that are traditionally based on agriculture. They are connected to a nationwide movement that grants social support to all its member communities. The Gaza perimeter is the area within Israel bordering the Gaza Strip.

References

Amit, K., & Fleischer, N. 2005, 'Between Social Resilience and Social Capital' in *The Concept of Social Resilience*, eds. N. Friedland, A. Arian, A. Kirschenbaum, K. Amit, & N. Fleischer, Samuel Neaman Institute, Forum of National Security, Society & National Security Program, Haifa, pp. 82–107. (Hebrew)

Arian, A., Nachmias, D., Navot, D., & Shani, D. 2003, 'The Israeli Democracy Index', Israel Democracy Institute, Guttman Center. Available from www.idi.org.il [11 July 2010]. (Hebrew)

Ben-Dor, G. 2003, 'Haifa Indicators—Task Force Report'. Fourth Herzliya Conference, Herzliya. Retrieved on 31 January 2010 from www.herzliyaconference.org/_Uploads/1028gabibendor.pdf

Ben-Dor, G., Canetti-Nissim, D., & Halperin, E. 2007, 'The Social Component of National Resilience', presentation given at the Seventh Herzliya Conference, Herzliya. Available from www.herzliyaconference.org/_Uploads/2805GabrielBenDor.ppt [20 January 2010]. (Hebrew)

Berger, R. 2007, 'The Abdication of Responsibility for Civilian Society by the Central Government during and in the Aftermath of Major Disasters', paper presented at the annual meeting of the Inter-University Seminar on Armed Forces Society, Chicago.

Berger, R., & Gelkopf, M. 2007, *The Effects of Ongoing Stress on Sderot and the Gaza Perimeter*, unpublished manuscript.

Bleich, A. 2000, 'Military Psychiatry in Israel: a 50-Year Perspective', *Harefuah*, vol. 138, no. 9, pp. 728–733.

Bleich, A. 2006, 'He Who Has a "Why" to Live for Can Bear Almost Any "How"', *BeNoge'a LaRegesh*, NATAL, Issue 8 (May). (Hebrew)

Bleich, A. 2007, 'Personal Resilience, Social Resilience', *BeNoge'a LaRegesh*, NATAL, Issue 9 (April). (Hebrew)

Cahlink, G. 2001, 'Defense Department Creates Civilian Purple Heart', *Government Executive*, 27 September.

Elran, M. 2006, 'Israel's National Resilience: the Influence of the Second Intifada on Israeli Society', Jaffee Center for Strategic Studies at Tel Aviv University, Memorandum No. 81, pp. 5–6 . (Hebrew)

Even, N. 2007, *Fallen Civilians: the Attitude of Governmental and Social Institutions toward Civilians Killed in Hostile and Terrorist Acts: Israel as a Test Case (1970–2000)*, doctoral dissertation, Bar-Ilan University. (Hebrew)

Friedland, N. 2005, 'The Elusive Concept of "Social Resilience"', Neaman Institute.

Friedman, A., Ben-Shalom, Y., Gal, J., Dahan, M., Lev-Sadeh, D., & Schmid, H. 2003, 'Report of the Cohesion and Social Resilience Team', presentation given at the Third Herzliya Conference, Herzliya. Available from www.herzliyaconference.org/_Uploads/1170socialstrength.pdf [11 July 2010].

Gal, R. 2003, 'National-Social Resilience: Behavioral and Cognitive Indices for Evaluating Israeli Societal Resilience vis-à-vis Terrorism during the Intifada', presentation given at the Third Herzliya Conference, Herzliya.

Karman, R., Tzur, Y., & Mendelovitch, Y. 2004, 'How We Became Bereaved Parents', *Walla News*, 26 April. (Hebrew)

Kasher, A. 2005, 'Collective Emotions, National Mourning and Terrorism' in *Mental Health in Terror's Shadow: the Israeli Experience*, eds. E. Somer & A. Bleich, Ramot, Tel Aviv, pp. 479–498. (Hebrew)

Kim, H. 1998, 'Between One Form of Bereavement and Another', *Haaretz*, 25 August. (Hebrew)

Klein, U. 2006, 'Who Is a Member of the Bereavement Family?', *Haaretz*, 2 May.

Lahad, M., Shacham, M., & Shacham, Y. 2010, 'The Impact of the Second Lebanon War on the Experience of Trauma and on the Resilience of Jews and Arabs in Northern Israel: a Longitudinal Study', in *Health, Education and Welfare Services in Times of Crisis: Lessons Learned from the Second Lebanon War*, eds. F. Azaiza, N. Nachmias, & M. Cohen, Pardes, Haifa, pp. 117–144. (Hebrew)

Lapid, Y. 2000, 'Not Final', *Maariv*, 5 May. (Hebrew)

Levy, A., Witztum, E., Granek, M., & Kotler, M. 1990, 'The Treatment of Combat Stress Reaction in the IDF, 1948–1973', *Harefuah*, vol. 32, pp. 49–53.

Mills, H., & Dombeck, M. 2005, *Resilience: Hardiness*. Available from www.mentalhelp.net/poc/view_doc.php?type=doc&id=5791&cn=209 [4 July 2010].

Mosse, G. 1990, *Fallen Soldiers: Reshaping the Memory of the World Wars*, Oxford University Press, New York.

Rein, L. 2011, 'Fallen Heroes Bill Honors 9/11 Victims', *Washington Post*, 27 December.

Shamai, M. 2010, 'Returning to Solidarity between the State and Its Citizens' in *Health, Education and Welfare Services in Times of Crisis: Lessons Learned from the Second Lebanon War*, eds. F. Azaiza, N. Nachmias, & M. Cohen, Pardes, Haifa, pp. 61–67. (Hebrew)

Tzur, Y. 2010, Speech at the memorial ceremony on Mount Herzl. Available from www.irgun.org.il/index.asp?PageCode=1 [3 July 2010]. (Hebrew)

Witztum, E., & Malkinson, R. 1993, 'Bereavement and Memorialization: the Two Faces of the National Myth' in *Loss and Bereavement in Jewish Society in Israel*, eds. E. Witztum & R. Malkinson, Kanah and the Ministry of Defense, Tel Aviv, pp. 231–258. (Hebrew)

Zigelman, Y., Shaham, M., Lahad, M., & Shaham, Y. n. d., *Developing Communal and Organizational Resilience via the Multidimensional Resilience Model*. Available from www.icspc.org/?CategoryID=164&ArticleID=120 [4 July 2010]. (Hebrew)

11 War Trauma in Israeli-Palestinian Society

> Suddenly I get a phone call . . . She says: You know a missile fell next to [. . .]'s house and people were killed? I immediately thought my child was killed because he's always hanging around the yard. I collapsed on floor . . . When I regained consciousness I cried and screamed, "My son is dead, my son is dead." In the meantime my brother called . . . He said it wasn't next to my house but next to . . . and that three young men were killed. Even though I understood what he said, I couldn't calm down. I constantly saw my son in front of my eyes. I don't know how I made it home . . . After that I couldn't think about anything else. I constantly envisioned my son before me in a horrific situation, dead or in a coffin or injured. I watched him all the time, I slept with him at night and held him . . . We aren't people who go to psychologists . . . But I went. I didn't tell anyone . . . I was afraid I was harming my son. I wanted to feel better . . . The psychologist helped me find strength . . . Now I'm all right. I let my son live his life.[1]

I decided to quote this lengthy portion of a conversation I had with a teacher in an Arab village in northern Israel in order to underscore the great similarity between Arabs and Jews in terms of the fear and sense of trauma that they experience during wartime. This should, theoretically, be obvious, yet Israeli Jews tend not to acknowledge the existence of such feelings within the Arab populace. Over the past decade, and particularly since the Second Lebanon War (2006), a certain interest has developed in war trauma among Arabs, though it has yet to penetrate Israeli public discourse. This inattention to Arab suffering reflects the prevailing view that Israeli Arabs are an alien minority that does not share the needs or security concerns of the general population and, instead, constitutes a burden and a threat. It also reflects discrimination against, and neglect of, an Arab population whose needs and problems elicit little interest. Although war trauma became a topic of public discourse among Jews only during the Al-Aqsa Intifada (2000–2004, also known as the Second Intifada), it has been addressed quite intensively and comprehensively since that time, from a myriad of perspectives. A similar development has yet to be seen regarding war trauma among Israel's Palestinian citizens.

Certain features of Israeli-Arabs' war trauma are reminiscent of the trauma experienced by Jewish-Israelis, while others are unique to the Arab community and arise from its status as a minority group that is discriminated against and subject to suspicions of hostility (Somer et al. 2005). In other words, in addition to the understandable fear of injury, death, or loss of loved ones, Israel's Arab citizens also have to cope with a lack of basic trust in their relationship with state authorities. To this, one may add the fact that the Jewish majority and the security forces suspect them of supporting hostilities against Jewish-Israelis, of rejoicing when such acts are committed, and even of cooperating with the perpetrators. Jewish society expects Israeli Arabs to publicly, immediately, and harshly denounce acts of terrorism, while not allowing them to condemn attacks on, or express solidarity with, Palestinians in the Occupied Territories. As noted in the report of the Or Commission, a commission of inquiry into the clashes between police forces and Israeli Arab citizens in October 2000 that marked the beginning of the Second Intifada, this state of affairs places Israel's Arab citizens in an emotional bind: they are caught between their sensitivity to, and identification with, the suffering of their fellow Palestinians and the fact of their Israeli citizenship.[2]

According to the Or Commission, the continual stress induced by this Catch-22 characterizes minority groups elsewhere in the world who live under inequitable social conditions in an atmosphere of racism, discrimination, and poverty.[3] In times of national emergency the severity of psychological trauma among such groups often exceeds that experienced by the majority population, particularly given the limited communal aid services and coping resources available to them. Discriminated minority groups tend to display low rates of participation in community emergency programs and generally prefer to rely on familial and social support networks, owing both to limited access to services and to the communal stigma attached to such external mechanisms (Somer et al. 2005). This pattern of behavior is found in Israel as well. Access to emotional support services in Arab localities is limited, as is the willingness to make use of these where they do exist. This unwillingness stems from a variety of causes, including cultural issues, the inferior quality of services available to Arabs, and fear of the community's disapproval should one seek assistance from the state (Levav et al. 2007).[4] Like other minority ethnic groups around the world, Israeli Arabs turn primarily to their neighbors in times of emergency. Seventy-two percent of them—three times the corresponding figure for Jews—feel duty-bound to help their neighbors in wartime (Lahad et al. 2010). This phenomenon should, presumably, indicate social cohesion, which itself promotes resilience. In this case, however, it appears to stem primarily from a lack of other support mechanisms, from the Arab localities' logistical unpreparedness for emergencies, from an overall sense of exclusion, and from a lack of faith in the availability of assistance from local and national authorities.

To all of the foregoing one may add the unprocessed trauma experienced by the Palestinian people as a whole, originating with the tragedy of 1948 (the Nakba, catastrophe in Arabic). Many villages were destroyed in the war, families divided, and hundreds of thousands of people uprooted from their homes. This experience is a focal point of unresolved pain within Palestinian collective memory, a tragedy that has never healed. The distress connected with the memory of the Nakba is likely intensified by the fact that the Israeli establishment—which views any commemoration of the event as a subversion of the Jewish narrative of Israel's founding, or even as an attempt to destroy the state from within—works to suppress it.[5] Most of the Israeli public also regards commemoration of the Nakba as an existential danger to Israel. In a survey that I conducted in June 2011 via Elixer Applied Research, 65% of the participants (64.58%) chose the most extreme degree of opposition (1 on a scale of 1 to 5) to Israeli recognition of the tragedy suffered by the Palestinian people in the wake of the War of Independence, or to any official expression of sympathy or empathy with the Palestinians in this regard, while only 5% felt that such recognition is crucial. Asked to explain their choices, the 65% who had unequivocally opposed recognizing the Nakba mounted the following arguments: the Palestinians were to blame for the disaster that they had suffered, since they were the ones who started the war (16%); that no such disaster had actually occurred (9%); that recognition would be a distortion of history (15%); and that recognition would lead to the State of Israel's destruction (10%).[6] As I have shown elsewhere (Keynan 2014), these findings have implications regarding Israeli emotional readiness for reconciliation. In the present context, however, they point to the extreme degree to which the collective Palestinian memory of trauma—a memory shared by Israel's Palestinian citizens—is being suppressed (ibid.).

Under these circumstances, it is hardly surprising that a research team led by Yitzhak Levav found higher rates of psychological disorder, including depression and anxiety, among Israeli Arabs than among Israeli Jews. They attribute this difference, in part, to rapid processes of social change that place modernity and tradition in daily conflict for Israeli Arabs, but also to the unprocessed trauma of the Nakba (Levav et al. 2007). Distinguishing between the effects of these two factors has yet to be systematically analyzed, but the aftereffects of displacement and collective loss, as manifested in emotional distress, have been demonstrated in other contexts, both Israeli and international. For example, a study of the reactions of the Jewish settlers of Gush Katif in the Gaza Strip, after their forced resettlement in Israel in 2005, found substantial emotional distress and demoralization. The risk factors for emotional distress typical of the Gush Katif evacuees have also been found among the Palestinians displaced in 1948, including feelings of alienation from the state and the sense that the sources of support provided by their now eradicated community were irreplaceable (Billig et al. 2006). The researchers attribute the reactions of Gush Katif evacuees to psychological processes of emotional closeness, an intimate familiarity and identification that produce attachment to a place (T. Fullilove, cited in Billig et al. 2006). Displacement, they argue, disrupts these processes and awakens nostalgia, confusion, and a sense of estrangement that manifest in emotional distress. There can be no doubt that the displacement and loss of the refugees exacerbate the emotional distress of war. The inability to talk about their trauma renders the emotional burden borne by Israel's Arab citizens all the more oppressive. This is a universal phenomenon familiar to trauma researchers, one that delays and, at times, prevents recovery (Herman 1994; LaCapra 2001). As such, it also increases the risk of becoming retraumatized in times of stress and crisis.

Israeli researchers first began to address psychological trauma among Israeli Arabs during the Al-Aqsa Intifada. Most of the findings were obtained through comparative studies of Jewish and Arab populations, calling attention to the broad distribution of psycho-trauma and high levels of fear within Israel's Arab society. Ben-Dor et al. (2007) find that during the four-year Intifada period, from October 2000 to October 2004, Arab-Israeli fear levels ranged from 4.41 at the beginning of the period to 4.15 at its end (on a scale of 1 to 6).[7] Although Jewish fear levels during this period were higher (4.73 to 5.19 on the same scale), when one considers that the Intifada-era terrorist attacks were directed primarily at the Jewish population, Arab fear levels appear particularly high. The level of emotional distress found among Arab adolescents after two years of terrorist attacks equaled that found among Jewish adolescents at the same point in time (Cohen et al. 2004).

These data are consistent with a pair of comparative studies that looked at the prevalence of PTSD symptoms throughout the Israeli population, 19 and 44 months after the outbreak of the Second Intifada. Although the Jewish sector, as noted earlier, was exposed to many more terrorist incidents than the Arab sector, these two populations exhibited no difference in stress- or PTSD-related symptoms at the 19-month point (Bleich et al. 2003). By the time of the second study at 44 months, stress- and PTSD-related symptoms had become more pronounced in the Arab sector (as well as among immigrants, women, and people with low levels of education) (Bleich et al. 2006). The study's authors attributed these findings to a dearth of services in the Arab sector. In other words, the erosion of resilience, experienced by all people when exposed to terrorism over extended periods, is exacerbated when resources are not available.

The paucity of services for Israel's Arab sector may be attributed to a combination of socio-geographic marginality and the prevailing perceptions of that sector as alien and hostile. Marginality is not unique to the Arab population, and the lack of social services and systemic support characterizes other marginal groups in Israel as well. However, the Jewish-Israeli perception of the Arab sector as a hostile and dangerous group exposes the latter to unique risk factors for stress and anxiety, the most obvious being the attitude of the security forces toward them.

The array of dangers with which Israeli Arabs are forced to contend can be glimpsed in the unfolding of the events of October 2000, the outbreak of the Second Intifada, and the subsequent wave of terrorism. Riots erupted in several Arab villages inside Israel, and Israeli security forces killed 12 Israeli Arabs and one non-Israeli Palestinian. The Or Commission's condemnation notwithstanding, the violence exhibited by the Israeli police toward the Arab demonstrators made it clear to Palestinian Israelis that their citizenship status is not equal to that of Jewish-Israelis, and that being Israeli citizens would not ensure their safety. A short time after these violent events the Second Intifada broke out, and the suicide attacks carried out on buses and public places took their toll on the Arab sector as well. Suad Suna Jabr, who was killed on board a bus at Karkur junction on the day she completed the final exams for her university degree (October 21, 2002); Minhal Dragma, who was killed in a terrorist attack while shopping at a market in Baka al-Sharkiya (February 21, 2002); Iman Kabha, killed on his way to the university while riding a bus in Jerusalem (June 18, 2002); Nawa Hinawi, killed in a terrorist attack while socializing with friends in a club in the Rishon LeZion industrial area (May 7, 2002)—all of these people, and other Arab citizens of Israel who lost their lives in terrorist attacks, exemplify the tragic shared fate of Arabs and Jews and demonstrate that Arab Israelis are indeed exposed to terrorism despite the fact that they tend not to live in those areas most frequently targeted.[8] However, this was not the view taken by Israeli Jews, and Israeli Arab society found itself in state of double distress: exposed to attacks by terrorists from outside Israel and to aggression and hostility on the part of the Israeli security forces and the Israeli state.

This phenomenon resurfaced during the Second Lebanon War in an even more distressing form. The total number of acute stress sufferers in the summer of 2006 was particularly high—1,900 according to National Insurance Institute data. Thousands of people experienced severe emotional stress that drove them to seek treatment. The high stress toll resulted from a lack of protective measures or emergency preparedness and from the nature of the attacks themselves: missile barrages that could not be adequately addressed by military means and that targeted city centers where no escape was possible; one was not safe even within the walls of one's home. The 3,970 missiles and shells that fell on Israel during the war had an impact similar to terrorism: the attacks disrupted the normal course of people's lives, and their time and location could not be predicted. Israeli citizens once again found themselves in conditions of increased risk for acute stress beyond that associated with natural disasters or other threats.

During the war some 20.3% of Israeli Arabs were found to suffer from acute stress, more than three times the corresponding figure for Israeli Jews (6.8%) (Cohen & Yahav 2010).[9] A month after the war, a study led by Mooli Lahad detected full-blown PTSD among Israeli Arabs in the areas under attack at twice the rate of Jews (41% versus 26% respectively). As the existing professional literature would have led one to expect, a repeat study conducted ten months after the war revealed a decline in PTSD within the population as a whole. Some of the trauma sufferers had recovered. Along with the general decline, the Jewish-Arab PTSD gap narrowed as well, but the Arab rate of incidence remained higher (30% compared with 23% for Jews) (Lahad et al. 2010).[10]

Trauma had a more profound impact on Arab society during the Second Lebanon War than during the Intifada period. Professor Khawla Abu-Baker presents instances of Arab men talking for the first time, toward the end of the war, about how trauma had affected them. Their statements evince a sense of helplessness, distress, and depression from fear of rocket attacks and the inability to protect their families (Abu-Baker 2006).

The general factors behind the high rates of acute stress and PTSD among Israeli civilians were exacerbated, as noted earlier, by factors unique to the Arab minority. The Second Lebanon War caught Palestinian Israelis even less prepared—physically and psychologically—than their Jewish counterparts. Many missiles fell in Arab areas and in the Arab neighborhoods of mixed cities, yet only in three of these places (Gush Halav, Fassuta, and Mi'ilya—areas that had been accorded "confrontation-line"[11] status in 1996) were residents briefed regarding any potential state of emergency. Most of the Arab localities had virtually no shelters or protected spaces, nor did they have any emergency services in place (Abu-Baker 2006). This state of affairs—the result of chronic and deep-rooted discrimination—reinforced the feeling among Arabs that state authorities neglected them. By contrast, as Lahad's study demonstrates, no significant difference existed between Jews and Arabs in their initial expectations of assistance from the local authorities and the government during the war. This kind of expectation is common among civilians in democratic countries, and the disappointment during the Second Lebanon War intensified the very feelings of fear and uncertainty that raise the risk of trauma. At the same time it further weakened the protective effects that come from faith in the availability of assistance when needed. Nevertheless, few Arab civilians left their areas of residence during the war, whether due to a lack of social ties in central Israel or due to cultural preference. Eighty-five percent of the Arab inhabitants of attack-prone areas remained in these areas throughout the war, as compared to just 33% of Jews (Lahad et al. 2010). This further eroded the Arabs' already-sparse coping resources.

During the Second Lebanon War the Arab localities came under direct attack for the first time in Israeli history. The injury rate in these areas was high, accounting for 40% of all Israeli fatalities (18 out of 44) (ibid.). Israeli Arabs had formerly believed themselves to be situated in a kind of no-man's land, beyond the reach of the Israeli-Arab conflict and unsusceptible to deliberate attack. This state of affairs collapsed without warning during the summer of 2006, and the difficulty of coping with the war became further complicated by a lack of emotional preparedness—yet another factor that research has shown to increase the risk of severe psychological distress (ibid.). Abu-Baker (2006) maintains that at the beginning of the war Palestinian Israelis believed they would not be targeted by Hezbollah and that any harm caused to them, whether physical or material, was due to error or bad luck. They blamed Israel for the war's outbreak and for the toll that the war imposed on them, even after hearing Nasrallah's admission of responsibility (and apology) for the deaths of two children—brothers Mahmoud and Rabia Taluzi of Nazareth.[12] However, Nasrallah's appeal to Haifa's Arab residents to leave the city in order to avoid injury was, in Abu-Baker's view, a threatening rather than a reassuring message. It even reawakened dormant, historically rooted feelings of distress. A similar appeal had been addressed to the parents of Haifa's Palestinian residents sixty years earlier: leave the city to ensure your safety. Nasrallah's appeal resurfaced the past experience of displacement and helplessness, and the unprocessed trauma of 1948.

Although Israel's Arab citizens would seem to exist outside the sphere of the Israeli-Palestinian conflict, they nevertheless experience a basic lack of security in their relations with the state: they fear confrontation with security forces and the enactment of unexpected and unjustified sanctions against them. The annual Index of Jewish-Arab Relations in Israel produced by Professor Sami Smooha of the University of Haifa points to the fact that a clear majority of Israeli Arabs fear major violations of their civil rights and even state violence or forced transfer.[13]

These feelings are understandable given certain incidents—exceptional though they may have been—in which Arab civilians were killed by the Israeli security forces, such as the Kafr Qasim massacre of 1956, the Land Day incidents of 1976, and the killing of 13 Arab demonstrators by the security forces in October 2000, as well as occasional, less-publicized events in which suspicion and hostility have been exhibited toward Arab citizens.

The 2006 Second Lebanon War exacerbated the already-tense relations between Jews and Arabs in Israel and showed that the wounds sustained in 2000 had yet to heal. The Jewish sector demanded that the Arab population unequivocally denounce the shelling of Israeli targets; it even expected, given the many Arab casualties, that Palestinian citizens of Israel would begin to exhibit a sense of partnership and shared destiny with the Jewish majority in the face of Hezbollah (Rekhess 2006). However, the Second Lebanon War proved yet another occasion in which Israeli Arabs found themselves caught between the demand that they condemn acts of hostility against Israel and the prohibition imposed on them by Israeli society against denouncing attacks on their fellow Palestinians—a dilemma already highlighted in 2000 by the Or Commission. Moreover, in the eyes of some Israeli Arabs, Hezbollah is not a terrorist organization but rather a "protest" movement, seeking to curb Israeli militarism and achieve a just end to the Israeli-Palestinian conflict. Due to all of these factors, Israeli Arabs rejected the demand that they openly take Israel's side (Samooha 2006). The Arabs also attributed the high number of Israeli-Arab fatalities to negligence on the part of the Israeli government, which had failed to provide them with shelters, warning systems, or protection. The Israeli public's harsh denunciation of statements made by Israeli Arab leaders regarding the war only intensified the Israeli-Arab dilemma of identity and deepened their sense of not belonging (Ben Caspit, quoted in Rekhess 2006). Arab alienation from the state has a domino effect that ultimately reinforces that very alienation—a sentiment that, during the Second Lebanon War, constituted yet another risk factor for psychological trauma. The lack of faith in the Israeli authorities directed Arab citizens toward Arab media sources, which portrayed Israel as the sole aggressor and broadcast unedited scenes of devastation and death in Lebanon. Televised images of this kind are known to increase anxiety, and they added to the frustration and sense of powerlessness experienced by Israel's Arab population (Abu-Baker 2006; Lahad et al. 2010).

Within this complex reality, Israeli Arabs are denied the opportunity to give meaning to their suffering and loss, one of the most important ways of coping with distress and bereavement. Their injuries and losses do not belong to dominant national narratives, whether Israeli or Palestinian, from which to draw reassurance or emotional resilience. Israeli Arabs have no share in the Jewish national ceremonies (except for the Druze and Bedouin, who serve in the IDF, and even for them participation is limited). No alternative ceremonial framework exists, given the complex and sensitive situation regarding Arab casualties by Palestinians as well as Jewish-Israeli suspicion of any Arab ceremony concerning the conflict as being defiance against the state. As one Palestinian-Israeli put it during the 2006 Lebanon War, "This war has once again placed us in a situation where we are uncomfortable with what is happening both to Israel and to the Arab countries" (quoted in Abu-Baker 2006, p. 11).

Israeli Jewish society pays little attention to war-related psychological trauma among the country's Arab population, a fact exemplified in certain processes undergone by the Israel Trauma Coalition (ITC) and NATAL (Israeli Center for Victims of War and Terror). In the wake of the Second Lebanon War the ITC, a coalition of several organizations working with victims of war trauma, decided to address the needs of the Arab Israeli population and created a unit to care for trauma in "special populations." The needs of immigrants, demobilized soldiers, and Gush Katif evacuees were already covered by ITC partner organizations (Sela, NATAL, and Mahut, respectively), while the Israeli-Arab sector had no organization capable of such care at the time (Friedman-Peleg 2008). The ITC therefore decided to establish a minorities' desk, a measure that, on the surface, reflected recognition of the deficit in Arab society and a commitment to address it. However, the decision to establish a minorities' desk, rather than creating a unit specifically for Israeli Arabs, demonstrated an emotional or conceptual barrier to acknowledging the legitimacy of Israeli-Arab suffering and psychological trauma and the difficulty in renouncing the exclusivity of Jewish suffering. In this sense, the ITC partner organizations reflect the inability of Israeli-Jewish society as a whole to call both Israeli Arabs and Palestinians by their names, employing, instead, the term "minorities." They also highlight the even greater inability of Jewish society to recognize that it is not alone in bearing the emotional and physical cost of the conflict and that it shares that burden with all of the other communities that live in the shadow of the conflict.

A similar difficulty to accept the existence of Arab war trauma and suffering could be seen in the process by which NATAL was established in 1998. The Hebrew name chosen by the organization's founders (*Nifge'ei Trauma al Reka Le'umi*—"Trauma Sufferers in a National Context") and the organization's symbol (the Israeli flag) proclaimed its status as a Jewish national organization committed to assisting Jewish trauma sufferers. This was a natural decision that accorded with the perspective of the Jewish majority, which viewed itself as the main, if not the only, casualty of the conflict. The symbol of the flag was later replaced with a tree, and the organization has recently begun seeking ways to assist trauma sufferers in the Arab sector, in a culturally sensitive manner.[14] However, the organization's very name, as well as its declared purpose of assisting those traumatized by the Israeli-Arab conflict, places it at the heart of the dilemma of Arab-Israeli identification.[15]

Israeli-Arab war trauma, with all of its unique features, is a topic that cries out for comprehensive future research. This chapter, which by no means encompasses the issue as a whole, is meant to underscore the Arab sector's status as a full-fledged component of Israeli society and of the home front that must be defended in wartime, as well as the great importance of including Israel's Arab citizens in the discourse of coping with war-related trauma. Such inclusion is important not only for Arab trauma sufferers as individuals but also for the essential role that an inclusive discourse might play in reshaping attitudes toward the conflict as a whole. As Professor Yolanda Gampel has noted, drawing on the work of Argentinean historian and sociologist Ignacio Lewkowicz, "Israelis and Palestinians bear a sense of immeasurable loss and endless mourning" (Gampel 2010, p. 156). So long as they remain unprocessed, the dark shadow of mourning and loss will continue to enshroud all parties to the conflict and prevent any escape from the cycle of bloodshed and trauma.

It is hardly surprising that there is so little awareness of the trauma suffered by Israel's Arab citizens. As noted in earlier chapters, war trauma is closely linked to national symbols and myths, meaning that any recognition of it entails confronting those symbols and myths and subjecting basic societal beliefs to scrutiny. Confrontation and scrutiny are difficult even when directed inward; they are significantly more problematic when related to a national minority perceived as hostile. To recognize the trauma of such a minority might blur the lines of justice and the distinction between aggressor and victim. In Israel, acknowledging that the Arabs also suffer war trauma involves defining them as casualties of the conflict and thereby redefining the way in which Jewish citizens perceive both the conflict and the Arabs themselves. As suggested by the findings of my survey on recognition of the Nakba, this kind of thinking generally arouses fear and ardent opposition. Any society in conflict would have trouble accommodating or accepting such an approach, and this is all the more true of Israeli-Jewish society, whose national identity is strongly marked by a history of suffering.[16] Yet recognizing war trauma of your adversaries is a revolutionary approach that delineates new boundaries for the identity of the conflict's victims, and if the parties to the conflict should succeed in adopting it, it could potentially serve as an impetus for reconciliation.

Notes

1. Confidential testimony delivered to the author, IK/NA, 14 July 2010.
2. Or Commission 2003, *Report of the State Commission of Inquiry regarding Clashes between the Security Forces and Israeli Citizens in October 2000*, http://brietman.homestead.com/vaadat-or/ [Hebrew]. The Or Commission was appointed by the Israeli government to investigate the events of October 2000 at the beginning of the Second Intifada in which 12 Arab citizens of Israel and one Palestinian were killed by Israeli police amid several demonstrations.
3. Ibid. The report quotes a special US government report prepared in the wake of 9/11.
4. The study was conducted in cooperation with the World Health Organization and the Israeli Ministry of Health. On the fear of disapproval see Yanay et al. (2005).
5. See a private bill approved by the Ministerial Committee for Legislative Affairs in May 2009, making it illegal to mark the Nakba as a day of mourning on Israeli Independence Day. The bill's explanatory section notes, "It is proposed that activities oriented toward marking Independence Day or the founding of the State as a day of mourning be prohibited, and that those who take advantage of the State of Israel's democratic and enlightened character—for the purpose of destroying it from within—be harshly punished." A softened version of the original bill was enacted into law by the Knesset, via the Budget Foundations Law (Amendment No. 40, 2011), but it retains the prohibition on marking Israeli Independence Day or the founding of the state as a day of

mourning. The law was passed on 22 March 2011. The bill and its explanatory material were published in *Knesset Bills*—315, 23 Adar 5770 (22 March 2011), p. 140. [Hebrew]

6. The survey was administered on 31 May–1 June 2011 to 508 adult Israeli Jews (age 18 and over), via an Internet panel. The interviewees constituted a random and representative sample of the adult Jewish-Israeli population that takes part in such panels (sampling error 4.35%). The questionnaire was prepared by the author in cooperation with Dr. Dorit Ben-Baruch, CEO of Elixer Applied Research. The questionnaire included items for which respondents had to rate their level of agreement/disagreement on a scale of 1 to 5, and an open question aimed at clarifying the reasons behind the ratings. The answers to the open question were subjected to text analysis, which assigned them to response clusters. A complete analysis of the survey and description of its methodology were published by the author in Keynan (2011).
7. The sample included Muslims, Christians, and Druze (see slide 40).
8. Data from a National Insurance Institute website dedicated to the memory of civilian victims of hostile acts. Retrieved 30 June 2011 from: http://laad.btl.gov.il/show_item.asp?itemId=39855&levelId=28553&itemType=10&template=3 [Hebrew].
9. The study was conducted in 2006.
10. The decline in the number of PTSD sufferers is consistent with Israeli findings from the Al-Aqsa Intifada period and with American findings from the period following 9/11—findings that point to reduced prevalence over time—and with the known fact that some patients succeed in recovering.
11. Areas that are considered especially dangerous based on their proximity to the border.
12. The two children, aged three and seven, were killed by a Katyusha rocket while playing in their backyard on 19 July 2006 (*NRG Maariv*, 21 July 2006).
13. The 2007 Index found that between 62% and 83% of Israeli Arabs fear major infringements of their civil rights—for example, state violence or transfer. In 2008 the Index showed that most Israeli Arabs (71.8%) fear infringements of their basic rights. The Index findings for the last few years may be viewed at Professor Sami Samooha's University of Haifa website: http://soc.haifa.ac.il/~s.smooha/page.php?pageId=166.
14. Among other things, NATAL has undertaken to identify an Arab sister organization with whom it might share knowledge and through which it might help Arab trauma sufferers. Announced at NATAL's annual public board meeting, February 2011.
15. NATAL website: www.natal.org.il/?CategoryID=162 [Hebrew].
16. On this topic see Keynan (2009).

References

Abu-Baker, K. 2006, 'Social and Psychological Coping on the Part of the Palestinian Family and Palestinian Society during the Second Lebanon War', *Inyan Mishpahti* [A family matter—bulletin of the Israel Association of Family Therapy], vol. 54, pp. 10–12. (Hebrew)

Ben-Dor, G., Canetti-Nissim, D., & Halperin, E. 2007, 'The Social Component of National Resilience', presentation given at the Seventh Herzliya Conference, Herzliya. Available from www.herzliyaconference.org/_Uploads/2805GabrielBenDor.ppt [20 January 2010]. (Hebrew)

Billig, M., Kohn, R., & Levav, I. 2006, 'Anticipatory Stress in the Population Facing Involuntary Removal in the Gaza Strip', *Journal of Nervous and Mental Disease*, vol. 194, no. 3, pp. 195–200.

Bleich, A., Gelkopf, M., Melamed, Y. & Solomon, Z. 2006, 'Mental Health and Resilience following 44 Months of Terrorism: a Survey of an Israeli National Representative Sample', *BMC Medicine*, vol. 4, p. 21.

Bleich, A., Gelkopf, M., & Solomon, Z. 2003, 'Exposure to Terrorism, Stress-Related Mental Health Symptoms, and Coping Behaviors among a Nationally Representative Sample in Israel', *JAMA*, vol. 290, pp. 612–620.

Cohen, M., Eid, J., & Haber, L. 2004, 'Responses of Arab and Jewish Adolescents to the Threat of Terrorism', *Society and Welfare*, vol. 24, no. 2, pp. 147–61. (Hebrew)

Cohen, M., & Yahav, R. 2010, 'Stress Reactions among Residents of Northern and Central Israel and among Jews and Arabs during the Second Lebanon War' in *Health, Education and Welfare Services in Times of Crisis: Lessons Learned from the Second Lebanon War*, eds. F. Azaiza, N. Nachmias, & M. Cohen, Pardes, Haifa, pp. 77–94. (Hebrew)

Friedman-Peleg, K. 2008, *The Nation on the Couch: the Use of Therapeutic Conceptualizations of Trauma and 'Resilience' in the Wake of the Al-Aqsa Intifada, the Disengagement and the Second Lebanon War*, doctoral dissertation, Tel Aviv University.

Gampel, Y. 2010, *The Parents Who Live through Me: the Children of War*, Keter, Jerusalem. (Hebrew)

Herman, J. L. 1994, *Trauma and Recovery*, Basic Books, New York.

Keynan, I. 2009, 'Collective Memory and Intergroup Leadership: Israel as a Case Study', in *Crossing the Divide: Intergroup Leadership in a World of Difference*, ed. T. L. Pittinsky, Harvard Business Press, Boston, pp. 219–230.

Keynan, I. 2011, 'The River of Forgetfulness: Collective Memory and Emotional Readiness for Reconciliation: Israel as a Case Study', paper presented at *International Journal of Arts and Sciences* (IJAS) & European Confederation of Upper Rhine Universities, Conference for Academic Disciplines, Aix-En-Provence, June.

Keynan, I. 2014, 'Between Past and Future: Persistent Conflicts, Collective Memory, and Reconciliation', *International Journal of Social Sciences*, vol. 3, no. 1, pp. 19–28.

LaCapra, D. 2001, *Writing History, Writing Trauma*, Johns Hopkins University Press, Baltimore.

Lahad, M., Shacham, M., & Shacham, Y. 2010, 'The Impact of the Second Lebanon War on the Experience of Trauma and on the Resilience of Jews and Arabs in Northern Israel: a Longitudinal Study', in *Health, Education and Welfare Services in Times of Crisis: Lessons Learned from the Second Lebanon War*, eds. F. Azaiza, N. Nachmias, & M. Cohen, Pardes, Haifa, pp. 117–144. (Hebrew)

Levav, I., Al-Krenawi, A., Ifrah, A., Geraisy, N., Grinshpoon, A., Khwaled, R., & Levinson, D. 2007, 'Common Mental Health Disorders among Arab-Israelis: Findings from the Israel National Health Survey', *Israel Journal of Psychiatry and Related Sciences*, vol. 44, no. 2, pp. 104–113.

Rekhess, E. (ed.) 2006, 'The Israeli Arabs and the War in the North', *Tmunat Matzav*, special edition, 14 August, the Moshe Dayan Center and the Konrad Adenauer Program for Jewish-Arab Cooperation. Available from www.dayan.org/kapjac/files/War_North1.pdf [1 April 2010]. (Hebrew)

Samooha, S. 2006, 'The Israeli Arabs and the Second Lebanon War', *Ofakim Hadashim Online*, vol. 33, 26 October. (Hebrew)

Somer, E., Or-Chen, K., & Peled-Avram, M. 2005, 'When My People Fight against My Country: Exposure to Terrorism, Distress and Coping among Israeli Arabs' in *Mental Health in Terror's Shadow: the Israeli Experience*, eds. E. Somer & A. Bleich, Ramot, Tel Aviv, pp. 77–110. (Hebrew)

Yanay, U., Prior, R., & Baer, S. 2005, *Victims of Hostile Acts in Israel: Injuries, Needs, Legislation and the Delivery of Services and Assistance*, School of Social Work, Hebrew University and the Research and Planning Authority, the National Insurance Institute, Jerusalem. (Hebrew)

Part III

The Shadow of War in People's Hearts

In Lieu of a Conclusion

12 The "Invention" of Trauma

Debate and Conceptualization

As the twenty-first century dawned, a different kind of war showed its face in the Western world, piercing the veil of security in which Americans and Europeans had been wrapped ever since the thunder of falling shells had passed to distant continents decades earlier. This new type of war, the war of terrorism, targeted civilians rather than soldiers on the battlefield. Its effects were different, but devastating nonetheless. The large numbers of civilians suffering acute stress reaction (ASR) and PTSD produced by the September 11 attacks in the US and the Al-Aqsa Intifada in Israel (2000–2004) could hardly fail to attract attention, as did the 2004 Madrid train bombing and the 2005 London underground bombing. The high trauma toll elicited mixed reactions: feelings of empathy as well as denial and skepticism regarding the veracity of the statistics—particularly those attesting to the traumatization of many people who had not themselves been present at the events.

Studies conducted in Israel and in the US between 2000 and 2004 identified a substantial presence of post-traumatic symptoms and even of full-blown PTSD outside the sites of the terrorist attacks.[1] These studies revealed mixed findings—while some found direct exposure to the terror attack to be a vital factor in the occurrence of PTSD (Neria et al. 2006), others found indirect exposure to be related to PTSD, despite physical distance from the site of the attack (Caspi 2003; Cohen Silver et al. 2002). While this raised questions regarding the findings' reliability and data collection methods, it also reignited the debate over how PTSD had been defined over the years in the *Diagnostic and Statistical Manual of Mental Disorders* published by the American Psychiatric Association (DSM), and the kinds of events thought to induce it. Critics restated earlier arguments against overly broad DSM criteria, particularly those that acknowledged the observation (through the media) of death or serious injury to others in the context of a violent attack or war as an event potentially causing PTSD (American Psychiatric Association 2000, especially Criterion A1).

The Al-Aqsa Intifada in Israel (2000–2004) and 9/11 in the US put the time-accepted PTSD definition (APA 2000) to a test in the context of unprecedentedly large-scale events that transposed the war-trauma debate from the battlefield, where most casualties are soldiers, to the civilian sphere—the soft underbelly of the democratic states. The debate was influenced—as always in trauma discourse—by nonscientific factors, including the fact that war-related PTSD in civilians was a new and little known experience, and the impact of the media seemed alternatively exaggerated or alarming. The multiple traumatic injuries among civilians were perceived as a threat to the social order and to national resilience. The professional disputes notwithstanding, this may have been the source of the harsh criticism directed at the broad DSM definition and consequent large-scale diagnosis of PTSD (inspiring the term "virtual epidemic") (Young 2007), which included individuals who had had indirect exposure to the events in question.

When analyzing the criticism, one has to take into account two unprecedented environmental features of the new format of war and the media: the attacks' staggering scope and unpredictability, which precluded any efforts to prepare for them, and the radical changes in global news reporting. September 11 was a milestone event that altered air travel habits and undermined the sense of security previously enjoyed by citizens of the Western world. The sheer extent of the damage, and the widespread astonishment at the ease with which thousands of civilians could be killed and injured in New York City's monumental towers, eroded feelings of security elsewhere as well. Suddenly, it seemed that nothing was immune to terror. Moreover, as Neria et al. (2006) showed, the WTC attack wiped out a whole community that worked and lived not only in the Twin Towers but also in their whole area. The traumatic implications of such a huge-scale disaster are naturally far more significant than the actual exposure to the attack.

In Israel, at the same time, the Al-Aqsa Intifada was raging: this was the second large-scale terrorist campaign to be launched in the space of a decade,[2] at a point when Gulf War–era fears of nonconventional weapons still lingered in public consciousness. The frequent terrorist attacks and their high death toll (see Chapter 8) awakened repressed fears of massive civilian targeting and weakened the sense of relative safety that the Israeli home front had formerly enjoyed. The occurrence of mass-casualty events in places geographically distant from each other intensified the impact of each event: the short intervals between them gave rise to a feeling that no place was safe, and that terrorists might strike anywhere, at any time.

The pervasive sense of fear was further aggravated by the far-reaching changes in local and global media. Scholars of the mass media note that the altered character of news reporting undermined viewers' sense of existential security. These scholars refer primarily to 24/7 news broadcasting as well as to the phenomenon of "breaking news"—the coverage of events as they occur—supported by technologies that make it possible to transmit information instantly from place to place, often unedited (Blondheim & Leibes 2009). In past years, when the news was presented in a regular time slot and in the authoritative voice of a dignified anchorperson, along with reassuring commentary, the newscast had a soothingly mediatory quality that conveyed that "someone was in charge," however frightening the circumstances. Naturally, this kind of news had its shortcomings, mostly of broadcasting a closed narrative, but its reassurance advantage is absent in the new genre, when we are inundated with direct, uncensored information that is virtually unavoidable. Increasingly, over the last two decades, information is disseminated, replicated, and broadcast repeatedly via all existing media outlets, which themselves strive to secure viewership ratings by offering the crudest and most sensational images and information. The aggressive invasion of unfiltered information into private space, combined with the actual threat posed by terrorism, had a profoundly deleterious effect on citizens' perceived existential security. These developments may partially explain the high incidence of post-traumatic symptoms even in people who had not been directly exposed to danger, and may even justify the broad PTSD definition in DSM-IV.

Such explanations of the overwhelming spread of PTSD, however, did nothing to dispel the idea of an "epidemic" being underway, nor did they quell doubts as to the reliability of the PTSD statistics or the validity of the original definition. In addition, the intensified exploitation of PTSD, which was thrust into daily use, as well as in the service of unrelated agendas, fostered distrust and even contempt. In recent years, PTSD has become raw material for biased, unreliable film and television representations, and employed as an excuse for criminality, violence, and antisocial behavior.[3] Thus, growing awareness of PTSD has actually intensified public disdain and, by extension, reinforced earlier criticism of "overly indulgent" definitions of the disorder's criteria or triggers (Young 2007). As a result, voices called to turn the clock back slightly on recognition of PTSD, mainly by narrowing the diagnostic criteria. The criteria were indeed changed in the next edition of DSM (APA 2013), which excluded emotional distress resulting from observation of a traumatic event through the media, and restricted the criterion to *witnessing in person*. On the other hand, the 2013 edition broadened the qualifying stressors (criterion A1), both by eliminating the DSM-IV A2 criterion of immediate response of fear, helplessness, or horror, and by adding criterion A4, which refers to repeated or extreme exposure to the aversive details of a traumatic event(s) (Levin et al. 2014). The few comparative studies that by now have explored the implications of the new definition did not show significant findings as to the impact of the new set of criteria. One such study (Stein et al. 2014) compared PTSD prevalence in 13 countries, according to DSM-IV, DSM-V, ICD-10, and ICD-11 (ICD- International Statistical Classification of Diseases and Related Health Problems, equivalent to DSM). The researches of this study conclude that the refinements in DSM-V are not associated with major changes in PTSD prevalence and that all four PTSD definitions offer information on unique, clinically significant cases that are omitted from the other manuals. Therefore, they advise using a broadened definition based on all four definitions. Calhoun et al. (cited in Levin et al. 2014), on the other hand, found more decisive findings and show that narrowing the indirect exposure criterion (A3) decreased PTSD diagnoses by 6% or 7%. It should be noted, though, that since only a short time has passed from the publication of the new DSM criteria, it is too early to judge its implications.

While these implications are still arguable, it is quite agreed that DSM-V improved the definition by eliminating criterion A2 of the previous edition, which requires an immediate response of intense fear, helplessness, or horror. Scholars now agree that this is not scientifically predictive of PTSD, and that army personnel, for example, are trained to conceal such feelings (ibid.). Another important contribution of DSM-V is the decision to separate it from the anxiety classification and include it in a new chapter on trauma and stressor-related disorders.

Awareness of the bloodless wounds sustained by combatants and by civilians has come full circle from denial to recognition to partial denial. The partial regression in accepting trauma is seeping through the cracks of doubts still lingering in many people's minds. The voices of denial may—by now—accept the actual existence of PTSD but go back to doubt its prevalence, still attempting to portray it as an overblown societal invention (Bracken 1998; Bryant & Harvey 2000; McNally et al. 2003; Summerfield 2001). Even supporters of the injury's existence have recently spoken out against the inflated use of the terms "trauma" and "post-trauma," which they believe has grown out of all proportion (Neuner 2009). This vacillation between recognition and nonrecognition is closely related to the political and social implications of the psychological trauma. As has been noted throughout this book, war-related psychological trauma has never been a matter for dispassionate assessment. Its invisibility—the fact of it being a hidden wound in the heart of its sufferers—eludes the simple, direct manner of comprehension as in physical injury. Open to interpretation, psychological trauma stands at the center of professional, economic, and political debates, and is appropriated in the service of national symbols and myths.

The inclusion of PTSD in the DSM and its representation as a direct result of violent external events—one that can afflict soldiers in wartime in the absence of any preexisting psychological problems—occurred in a turbulent period in American history, as the US reeled from its involvement in the controversial Vietnam War. Opponents argued that the very inclusion of PTSD and its defining criteria resulted from political pressure and attempts to soften the hostile reception to American Vietnam veterans.[4] Refutations of this argument were mounted by many scholars, who insisted that the professional knowledge necessary for recognition of PTSD had already existed in the early 1970s, and that the political pressure by war objectors caused the decade-long delay in recognition, and not the other way around (Blank 1985). These latter researchers claimed that nonrecognition had been entwined with the American public's distaste for the war—aversion that was channeled into a sense of alienation and anger toward the veterans. The hostility veterans encountered was allegedly so ubiquitous as to prevent many veterans from talking about their experiences, even with their friends and families, as they found themselves bombarded with derogatory epithets ("child killers"). Overall, the Vietnam War aroused particularly strong emotions in the US, and the reactions of clinicians and therapists were likewise affected. For example, a 1984 psychiatric review article dismissed as marginal the role of war experiences in laying the foundations for PTSD in Vietnam veterans, and placed the responsibility for their adjustment difficulties on the veterans themselves, whom the author accused of being troublesome burdens to society from time immemorial (ibid.). This opinion echoes a situation that has persisted for centuries. Society sends soldiers to sacrifice their lives for ideals that it defines for them. Societies glorify heroism under fire and the willingness to go to war, and view such traits as societal values of the first order. Yet in too many instances, and no matter how subtle or well-disguised their efforts, these same societies deny responsibility for the fate of those who return wounded, and distance themselves from them.

In Israel, the professional approach to war trauma has similarly been subject to political, social, and ideological interpretations by clinicians and therapists, whose views are accorded particular importance due to their first-hand interaction with the wounded. Most of these professionals are careful to avoid pronouncements that might be interpreted as political judgments of the Israel-Palestinian conflict, and very rarely speak in public on how the country's military-political circumstances affect the mental health of soldiers or civilians. In fact, such careful avoidance is very much in line with Israeli society's political and ideological attitude toward war trauma. Warnings by senior psychologists that violent confrontation with the civilian Palestinian population might have harmful psychological effects on soldiers were construed as attempts to bring politics to bear upon military decision making (see Chapter 5); the hostile reception that these psychologists received from the defense establishment guaranteed that few would publicly voice their criticism.[5] Most therapists publically align with what they interpret as the Israeli consensus, maintaining that any other choice would be inappropriate politicization of their therapeutic work and, as such, would undermine their ability to offer treatment to all those in need.[6] However, a review of studies published by Israeli trauma researchers in local and international venues illustrates that this stance forces therapists into a political trap. Adamant refusal to discuss anything that might be seen as lying outside of the consensus is, after all, a political statement in itself. Historian José Brunner has shown that, in the Al-Aqsa Intifada period, professional-therapeutic engagement with trauma constituted, albeit unwittingly, an ideological statement, inasmuch as it remained solely within the bounds of the Jewish societal "consensus" and virtually never addressed the existence of war trauma on the Palestinian side (Brunner 2006). By restricting themselves, even unintentionally, to the "consensus," some cases of trauma are acknowledged while others are ignored, causing undertreatment of some trauma casualties. Since any engagement with Palestinian war trauma or with the trauma suffered by Israel Defense Forces (IDF) soldiers due to engagement with civilians is generally thought to reflect a political stance, it therefore arouses the establishment's distrust or outright disapproval and results in undertreatment. On the other hand, trauma suffered by Jewish settlers in the occupied territories,[7] even when triggered by violent confrontation with IDF soldiers or with police, is usually considered as a matter for routine clinical intervention. The situation is not irreversible. Whether clinical involvement with one kind of trauma should be regarded as "political" or "apolitical" depends entirely on one's point of view, or, to use the words of anthropologist Allan Young, PTSD is constituted of different epistemic cultures (Duclos 2013).

The politics of trauma is reflected in economic considerations as well: in particular, a desire to limit eligibility for disability benefits, as exemplified in the congressional decision concerning trauma casualties after 9/11. The congressional decision excluded PTSD sufferers from the circle of compensation (apart from funding for a short course of psychotherapy), unless they could also prove physical injury. The congress openly based the decision on their wish to minimize the compensation payable by insurance companies and the government. In a similar vein, US courts began to adopt a restrictive approach toward the recognition of PTSD among disabled war veterans, in stark contrast to the American Psychiatric Association's expansive approach.[8]

In Israel, the Goren Committee deliberation protocols[9] show a debate on the extent of the state's responsibility for war and security casualties, based also on economic considerations. The disagreements in the deliberations reflected financial and ideological differences, and echoed prevailing attitudes regarding the national importance of emphasizing the unique status of combat soldiers, ideological differences concerning the limits of the state's responsibility for its agents, and uncertainty regarding the definition of an agent of the state. The deliberations also give expression to conflicting views on the heroism/sacrifice ethos and its commemoration, as well as to concerns over potential devaluation of the terms "disabled IDF veteran" and "disabled veteran of the [other] security forces." More than anything else, the debates reveal the omnipresent sociocultural hierarchy that ranks the injured and the fallen by type and circumstances of injury, and relegates traumatized combatants to inferior status, compared to the physically wounded, even when both were injured in the same event. Statements by Brigadier General Avigdor Kahalani, for example, a decorated and highly admired war hero, to the Goren Committee (quoted in Chapter 4) reflect a pervasive tendency to dismiss the severity of psychological trauma. According to Kahalani, trauma is a routine experience for combat soldiers. "Every soldier who has fought on the battlefield has PTSD [. . .] Show me one combatant who doesn't have PTSD," he said, failing to comprehend the difference between painful memories of battle and traumatic injury.[10]

Such lack of comprehension is perpetuated by the insistence of the psychiatric establishment on the conceptualization of PTSD as a mental disorder instead of an injury, despite the understanding that trauma is caused by an external factor. Only recently, the American Psychiatric Association declined a request by American military leaders to change the name of the phenomena from disorder (PTSD) to injury (PTSI) (APA 2013). I expand on this issue elsewhere (Keynan 2014), but it is important to emphasize here the relevance of this debate to the full legitimization of trauma.

Despite the foregoing disputes, even the harshest critics of the DSM's PTSD definition and its adoption by the psychiatric establishment do not deny the existence of the symptoms that characterize the disorder. As noted by Allan Young, a leading opponent of the DSM definition since 1980, "The suffering is real. PTSD is real" (Young 1995, p. 10). The critics are not seeking to abolish recognition of the disorder; rather, they are trying to restrict its meaning and the kinds of events identified as precipitators of it.

On the other side of the divide are those who maintain that an overly narrow definition also has undeniable implications. American and Israeli studies point to the large numbers of demobilized soldiers who have never been diagnosed and have never sought assistance or therapy. These studies have called attention to accompanying disorders that are not included in the definition of PTSD, and to cases in which soldiers suffering distress and functional impairment identical to those of full-blown PTSD are not recognized as wounded veterans because their symptoms do not meet the disorder's precise clinical definition.[11] Moreover, post-traumatic impairment evolves and extends its reach over the years, and "metastasizes" to additional areas (Levin et al. 2014) "like a cancer of the soul,"[12] causing impaired memory and concentration, somatic symptoms, outbursts of anger, difficulty in controlling aggressive impulses, and more. Because this is an area where psychiatry converges with legal-economic practices, and a DSM-based psychiatrist's diagnosis is a basic condition of official recognition and eligibility for treatment and benefits, many veterans are not only denied appropriate recognition but also blamed for overstating or even faking their symptoms in order to receive benefits.

No less glaring a deficiency of the existing PTSD definition relates to the syndrome's social context, rooted in its centripetal (from the outside in) and centrifugal (from the inside out) features of trauma, as described by Kai Erikson (Erikson 1995), which doom the traumatized to prolonged and increasing alienation and irreversibly unravel their interpersonal relationships. Traumatized people feel impelled to isolate themselves from others and to withdraw from society. Preoccupied with denying their trauma, they retreat into a protective shell where they may feel more secure, but nevertheless suffer isolation and loneliness and experience a desire for human warmth, understanding, and acceptance. However, because these two desires cannot be satisfied simultaneously, a negative interaction emerges between PTSD casualties and those around them—one that exacerbates the vicious cycle of avoidance/attraction to interpersonal engagement. The outcome is a shattering of the traumatized individual's sense of intimacy with his immediate family and with his broader social environment.

These social implications of psychological trauma are usually regarded as less important from a medical-functional point of view—the main perspective from which the relevant authorities assess patient status. Moreover, functioning is generally measured in narrow terms that relate primarily to the patient's ability to hold a job and integrate into what is considered "normal" community life. Unfortunately, such a measurement approach reflects the inability of the general society to accommodate the internal contradiction posed by individual functioning that is simultaneously impaired and unimpaired.[13] This situation also underscores the Gordian knot entangling psychological trauma's medical-social definition and the unambiguous legal-economic criteria that are used to clearly distinguish between afflicted and healthy individuals.

Many trauma sufferers manage to function well at work, however ravaged their emotional lives may be. They divert all of their emotional energies to the task of functioning well on the job, and deplete the mental resources they need for normal interactions at the familial and social levels. Many mask their emotional dysfunction and loss of self by becoming workaholics. This kind of behavior can be a symptom of repressed and untreated injury, which is liable to worsen over the years, especially at points of career transition, or retirement, when the ego weakens. When the veil of normalcy is removed and these individuals are forced to confront the abyss they have struggled to avoid, they may sink into a personal crisis of catastrophic proportions.[14]

This issue has been somewhat addressed in DSM-V, which expanded DSM-IV criterion F, which spoke about "significant distress or functional impairment." What is now criterion G is phrased "clinically significant distress or impairment in social, occupation, or other important areas of functioning." It remains to be seen, however, how this phrasing will help clinicians comprehend the overall suffering PTSD creates, and find new ways to help casualties and their families.

There is little substance to the arguments that trauma is an overblown societal invention. These arguments appear to confuse popular/political discourse and erroneous findings with the fact that war trauma is a wound of the most devastating kind, accompanied by variable and complex manifestations. From a medical perspective, the "societal-invention" camp rejects that PTSD symptoms may include such complementary and accompanying disturbances as anxiety and depression, and disregards the tendency of psychological trauma to evolve over the years and spread to other parts of the psyche. Using functional arguments, the societal-invention camp emphasizes measurable, visible, easily identifiable symptoms that mesh with the prevailing socioeconomic agenda. This emphasis is exemplified by the preoccupation with employment and the concomitant disregard of impaired emotional functioning and of the irrevocable harm that trauma causes to its sufferers' interpersonal relations with their primary support base—their families and loved ones. This approach dooms trauma sufferers to the loss of their emotional lives, to unremitting loneliness even in the presence of those closest to them, and to deep, persistent distress.

Overemphasis on the technical components of the PTSD definition and statistics of incidence and prevalence conceals the real challenge: conceptualizing war trauma. This is more formidable a task than any posed by diagnostic obstacles, and is closely linked to a disinclination to openly discuss the macro-social effects of war itself. In this sense, the psychiatric definition of trauma trivializes the misery and horror produced by war. It turns that misery into a technical and medical issue (Summerfield 2001) and precludes discussion of the broader, universal experience of social suffering (Kienzler 2008) and the boundless sorrow that war imposes on all its unfortunate victims and their loved ones and family members. Ultimately, the conceptualization of war trauma should be more than a dry determination of disability ratings: it should recognize the multidisciplinary social and philosophical ramifications, as well as its medical symptomology. Limiting the discussion to technical matters suppresses the underlying issue and masks the human and social meaning of war itself.

Trauma has many forms, and many of the phenomena described here are common to all of them. Yet, *war trauma* has distinctive features shaped by its context of personal injury inflicted because of affiliation with the collective, via events that are national in character. From a diagnostic perspective, Hunt (2010) argues that although war trauma symptoms differ from one person to the other, most inflicted individuals share comorbid symptoms usually related directly to their particular role within the war they were part of, and therefore the medical model of mental disorders justifies the separation of war trauma from the PTSD classification all together. From a social perspective, the unique context of war trauma has contradictory implications for society. The collective context makes it difficult for society to grant legitimacy to the injured. It raises the specters of frailty, impaired fighting capability, and military powerlessness in the face of existing threats, and risks of diminished civilian morale and resilience. It also arouses concerns that the collective sense of justice will be undermined, in those instances where the traumatic event bears traces of inappropriate conduct. At the same time, however, the traumatized need this very legitimacy for their recovery process, which is closely linked to social recognition of their injury and the sacrifice they have made for others, precisely because their injuries are inseparably related to their societal affiliation. They, who are paying the price, desire recognition and devote much energy to a quest for social support and a warm national embrace and reciprocity in their relations with the state. Those who have sacrificed their well-being on behalf of the collective and have been changed forever by their sacrifice expect the nation to repay them in kind and to love and support them unconditionally. When the establishment is hesitant to respond—or, worse, when it denies or is mistrustful of their experience, trauma-wounded individuals feel betrayed and forsaken, and their already-sparse coping resources are depleted to an even more perilous degree.

The conflict between what traumatized individuals need and what society is willing to give them also spills over to healthy individuals, who experience guilt over the fate of those who have paid the price on the collective's behalf, but find it difficult to accommodate or fully understand the horrors to which the injured bear witness. The healthy members of society are torn between a sense of obligation toward those who have made a sacrifice and an ungovernable desire to put the injured and their suffering out of mind by disclaiming any responsibility for their fate. The result is a continual battle between recognition and denial, between knowing and not-knowing, between speaking and not-speaking. This struggle broadens the abyss between those who have paid the price and observers on the sidelines, and reinforces the latter's tendency to downplay the suffering of the former to assuage their own sense of guilt.

Notes

1. On Israel and the US, see Chapter 10, this volume. On Great Britain, see Rubin et al. (2005).
2. The earlier campaign was launched during the negotiations on the Oslo Accords by Palestinian extremists, who objected to the peace process.
3. Action-series heroes, demobilized soldiers, and civilians are frequently portrayed as PTSD sufferers whose disorder legitimizes their inappropriate behavior. See also Young (2007).
4. This argument is based on the fact that legislation had been needed in order to bring about the establishment of counseling centers for Vietnam veterans suffering from

myriad adjustment problems, including PTSD, after a decade of opposition on the part of the Veterans Administration (Summerfield 2001; Young 2002).

5. On clinician attitudes toward transparent trauma and its sufferers, see Chapter 5, this volume.
6. Bleich interview, 2009.
7. The Occupied Territories are the territories conquered by Israel in 1967, in the West Bank (also known as Judea and Samaria) and before 2005 also the Gaza Strip, from which Israel withdrew on that year.
8. On the courts' restrictive approach and the congressional decision, see Rimmerman et al. (2007, pp. 63–64). On the APA's approach, see APA (2000).
9. The Goren Committee was a public committee to examine eligibility for assistance from the rehabilitation divisions established by the government in May 2009. The committee was to formulate criteria for the circumstances under which the wounded and the families of fallen soldiers would be entitled to Defense Ministry support and assistance.
10. The Goren Committee, Statement of Avigdor Kahalani, 2010.
11. On the number of American veterans of service in Iraq and Afghanistan who suffer post-traumatic distress but whose injury is not recognized, see Rand (2008) and note 23 of Chapter 4, this volume. See also the recent report by an American congressionally mandated Institute of Medicine panel that estimates the numbers of American veterans seeking PTSD care as 500,000 (Thompson 2014). On the phenomenon in Israel, see data presented by Professor Zahava Solomon to the Goren Committee, pointing to high absolute numbers of undiagnosed trauma sufferers; also, Bleich and Solomon (2002); Goren Committee deliberations, Knobler testimony, p. 11.
12. Expression and description of Professor Zahava Solomon, Goren Committee deliberations, p. 3.
13. Barnea interview, April 2011.
14. Barnea interview, April 2011.

References

American Psychiatric Association 2000, *Diagnostic and Statistical Manual of Mental Disorders*, 4th edn., Washington D.C.

American Psychiatric Association 2013, *Diagnostic and Statistical Manual of Mental Disorders*, 5th edn. Available from www.dsm5.org.

Blank, A. S. 1985, 'Irrational Reactions to Post-Traumatic Stress Disorder and Viet Nam Veterans' in *The Trauma of War: Stress and Recovery in Viet Nam*, eds. S. M. Sonnenberg & A. S. Blank, American Psychiatric Press, Washington, DC, pp. 69–98.

Bleich, A., & Solomon, Z. 2002, 'Psychiatric Assessment of Mental Disability among PTSD Sufferers in the Defense System' in *Mental Disability: Medical, Research, Social, Legal and Rehabilitative Aspects*, eds. A. Bleich & Z. Solomon, Ministry of Defense, Tel Aviv, pp. 43–71.

Blondheim, M., & Leibes, T. 2009, 'Television News and the Nation: the End?', *ANNALS of the American Academy of Political and Social Science*, vol. 625, no. 1, pp. 182–195.

Bracken, P. J. 1998, 'Hidden Agendas: Deconstructing Post-Traumatic Stress Disorder,' in *Rethinking the Trauma of War*, eds. P. J. Bracken & C. Petty, Free Association Books, New York, pp. 38–59.

Brunner, J. 2006, 'The Never-Ending Story: Trauma and Ideology in the Shadow of the Al-Aqsa Intifada', *Theory and Criticism*, vol. 28, pp. 231–239. (Hebrew)

Bryant, R. A., & Harvey, A. G. 2000, 'New DSM-IV Diagnosis of Acute Stress Disorder', *American Journal of Psychiatry*, vol. 157, pp. 1889–1890.

Caspi, M. 2003, Research and Information Center, the Knesset, background document for deliberations on the topic of terrorism-related anxiety among children. Available from www.knesset.gov.il/mmm/data/pdf/m00608.pdf.

Cohen Silver, R., Holman, A. E., McIntosh, D. N., Poulin, M., & Gil-Rivas, V. 2002, 'Nationwide Longitudinal Study of Psychological Responses to September 11', *JAMA*, vol. 288, pp. 1235–1244.

Duclos, V. 2013, 'When Anthropology Meets Science: an Interview with Allan Young'. Available from http://somatosphere.net/2013/10/when-anthropology-meets-science-an-interview-with-allan-young.html [8 August 2014].

Erikson, K. T. 1995, 'Notes on Trauma and Community' in *Trauma: Explorations in Memory*, ed. C. Caruth, Johns Hopkins University Press, Baltimore, pp. 183–199.

Hunt, N. C. 2010, *Memory, War and Trauma*, Cambridge University Press, New York.

Keynan, I. 2014, 'Injury or Disorder? The Significance and Implications of War Trauma Terminology', *Society and Welfare, Social Work Quarterly*, forthcoming. (Hebrew)

Kienzler, H. 2008, 'Debating War-Trauma and Post-Traumatic Stress Disorder (PTSD) in an Interdisciplinary Arena', *Social Science & Medicine*, vol. 67, no. 2, pp. 218–227.

Levin, A. P., Kleinman, S. B., & Adler, J. S. 2014, 'DSM-5 and Posttraumatic Stress Disorder', *Journal of the American Academy of Psychiatry and the Law Online*, vol. 42, no. 2, pp. 146–158.

McNally, R. J., Bryant, R. A., & Ehlers, A. 2003, 'Does Early Psychological Intervention Promote Recovery from Posttraumatic Stress?', *Psychological Science in the Public Interest*, vol. 4, no. 2, pp. 45–79.

Neria, Y., Gross, R., & Marshall R. D. 2006, 'Mental Health in the Wake of Terrorism: Making Sense of Mass Casualty Trauma', in *9/11: Mental Health in the Wake of Terrorist Attacks*, eds. Y. Neria, R. Gross, & R. D. Marshall, Cambridge University Press, New York, pp. 3–14.

Neuner, S. 2009, Book review of A. Sarat, N. Davidovitch, & M. Albertstein (eds.) 2007, *Trauma and Memory: Reading, Healing and Making Law*, *Social History of Medicine*, vol. 22, no. 2, pp. 435–437.

Rand—Center of Military Health Policy Research 2008, 'Invisible Wounds of War'. Available from www.rand.org/content/dam/rand/pubs/monographs/2008/RAND_MG720.pdf.

Rimmerman, A., Tal-Katz, P., & Avrami, S. 2007, 'People Injured in Acts of Terror in Israel and the United states: a Comparative Review and Future Recommendations', *Social Security*, vol. 73, pp. 41–68. (Hebrew)

Rubin, G. J., Brewin, C. R., Greenberg, N., Simpson, J., & Wessely, S. 2005, 'Psychological and Behavioural Reactions to the Bombings in London on 7 July 2005: Cross Sectional Survey of a Representative Sample of Londoners', *British Medical Journal*, vol. 331, no. 7517, p. 606.

Stein, D. J., McLaughlin, K. A., Koenen, K. C., Atwoli, L., Friedman, M. J., Hill, E. D., & Maercker, A. 2014, 'DSM-5 AND ICD-11 Definitions of Posttraumatic Stress Disorder: Investigating "Narrow" and "Broad" Approaches', *Depression and Anxiety*, vol. 31, no. 6, pp. 494–505.

Summerfield, D. 2001, 'The Invention of Post-Traumatic Stress Disorder and the Social Usefulness of a Psychiatric Category', *British Medical Journal*, vol. 322, pp. 95–98.

Thompson, M. 2014, 'The PTSD Epidemics: Many Suffering, Few Solutions', *Time*, 24 June.

Young, A. 1995, *The Harmony of Illusions: Inventing Post-Traumatic Stress Disorder*, Princeton University Press, Princeton.

Young, A. 2002, 'The Self-Traumatized Perpetrator as a "Transient Mental Illness"', *L'Évolution Psychiatrique*, 67, pp. 630–650.

Young, A. 2007, '9/11: Mental Health in the Wake of Terrorist Attacks', *Journal of Nervous and Mental Disease*, vol. 195, no. 12, p. 1030.

13 From Stone to Lake and Back

The Individual and Collective Circles of Trauma

Trauma has a certain ripple effect, similar to that observed when a stone is thrown into a lake. Trauma affects not only the individuals afflicted with it but also their spouse and children; entire families can suffer from what is known in the literature as secondary trauma (Solomon et al. 1992). Extending outward in ever-widening circles, the repercussions of trauma reach the entire national community, and the scars borne by individuals can merge into a whole that is greater than the sum of the suffering individuals, producing a group ethos that bears the hallmarks of trauma (Erikson 1995).

There is a close relationship between the personal stories of trauma casualties and the overarching story of their national group, and this phenomenon is especially pronounced in societies like Israel that bear the memory of past collective trauma and are also mired in a current protracted conflict. The historical continuum from the traumatic national past to the contemporary conflict fuels a vicious cycle: the collective memory justifies pursuing the conflict, while the conflict engenders yet another menacing collective memory, and so on. In a never-ending process, representations of the distant past blend with the continually emerging live memory. The new narratives of pain that are constantly being written connect with the traumatic national history, some of whose survivors still live, and together they inundate the psyche with existential fears and doubts over the possibility of ever escaping the cycle of violence and terror. The way the war fallen are remembered and honored also infuses personal stories with collective overtones, in a reciprocal manner: the plane of personal mourning is shaped by social forces and cultural values, while the modes of collective commemoration are influenced by the attitudes and demands of bereaved individuals (Bilu & Witztum 2000).

Israeli society behaves as though caught in a vise between the overwhelming traumatic memory of the Holocaust, on the one hand, and the consequences of the current conflict, on the other hand. The traumatic memory of the Holocaust has shaped the entire national mode of thought and conduct, while at the same time, the lives of tens of thousands of individuals and their families bear the ongoing effects of the Israeli-Palestinian conflict, having been seemingly selected to pay the price of their national affiliation on behalf of the entire group. Israel is a small country, and the number of those injured in some way or another as a result of the Israeli-Palestinian conflict is so large that nearly every individual has been injured or knows someone who was directly or indirectly harmed.[1] When to this number we add the population of Holocaust survivors and their families,[2] we obtain the wretched picture of "a near infinity of private sorrows,"[3] a mingling of personal and collective traumatic memories that permeate the shared experience to create a unique kind of cultural identity (Nora 1989).

This is the shadow of war in people's hearts: a trauma ethos that draws one to envelope oneself in the shared purifying sorrow that erects walls of apathy and blindness toward similar emotions among other groups, and that leads to predetermined patterns of behavior; a self-fulfilling prophecy of impasse that repeatedly intercepts Israel's chances of normalization, both at the domestic level and in its relations with the outside world.

In a certain sense, one can think of collective trauma[4] as a kind of societal PTSD that strikes an entire community and affects all of its members (Eliot et al. 2004). The national psyche is not, of course, identical to the individual psyche, but the concepts relevant to individual trauma offer a conceptual framework that is valuable for the analysis of sociopolitical processes.[5] Like individual trauma, collective trauma undermines society's sense of stability and identity, and perpetuates feelings of endangerment, disorder, and profound fracture (Bodnar 1998). Paradoxically, despite the multiple individual traumas that make up the collective trauma, individual catastrophe pales in comparison with the overall destruction of the social or national fabric, and is often wholly eclipsed by the expectation that individuals should put aside their personal suffering and mobilize their emotional and other resources to ensure the survival of the shared collective framework. This may be nothing more than a natural protective mechanism of society, triggered by panic when the survivors of a collective trauma realize that their community is no longer their source of support, and that an important part of their own identity has disappeared along with the fragmentation of their society's identity (Erikson 1978; Neal 1998). This mechanism, however, causes grave injustice to those individuals who have been injured and are unable to muster their strength to reinforce collective resilience. The effects of this mechanism are particularly noticeable in Israeli society's ambivalent attitude toward Holocaust survivors, who—for many years—were perceived as having failed to defend either themselves or the nation, and as having gone like sheep to slaughter. Another, no less problematic effect of this mechanism is the entrenchment in misguided attitudes that lead to a fruitless quest for a sense of security and protection—an ever-elusive end that nonetheless seems to justify virtually all means.

The vicissitudes that have characterized Israeli society's approach to war trauma reveal, first and foremost, that as a collective, Israelis are motivated by profound fear, coupled with a deep desire to feel that their cause and their actions are not only justified but also just, even in cases when that feeling is deceptive. This fear-and-justice loop in which they are caught is itself the primary driver of their attitude toward war trauma. The fear accounts for old Israeli attitudes toward trauma casualties: alienation toward soldiers afflicted with combat stress reaction (CSR) during the War of Independence and their stigmatization as cowards and shirkers;

a gnawing fear that war trauma heralds a decline in civilian fortitude; and a growing tendency to view the current legitimization of trauma as disproportionate or excessive. As I have shown earlier (Chapter 5), the yearning to be morally right is reflected in the refusal to recognize moral injury, trauma suffered by soldiers in situations of harmful military activity within a civilian population (Shay 2010). Struggling to maintain their conviction in Israel's moral superiority, many Israelis tend to not to assess such events objectively, but rather via a political prism, shaped by the need for moral reassurance, often dismissing the information as false attempts to harm the IDF's reputation. This same subjugating motivation lies behind Jewish-Israelis' disregard of the war trauma experienced by Palestinians, whether they are residents of Gaza and the West Bank or Israeli citizens. Awareness of Palestinian trauma is forcibly repressed because its recognition might raise doubts as to the solidity of the imagined boundary dividing those whom Israel believes to be persecuted from those believed to be the persecutors, between the just and the guilty.

The motivation of fear and the motivation of rightness are linked as variables in an equation that demands fortitude and unquestioned faith in the justice of Israel's cause, in all situations. This equation has dominated Israeli discourse for many years, and may partly explain the inner contradiction that characterizes large segments of Israeli society—a nation whose public life is so thoroughly permeated by an experience of shared suffering yet expresses suspicion and insusceptibility toward individual suffering, and finds it so hard to feel empathy toward the suffering of other nations.[6] During the War of Independence this overpowering ring of fear and justice functioned as a social defense mechanism against the dreadful apprehensions of defeat and of losing the as-yet unborn state, in a period when even physicians believed in the fortifying power of patriotism and of conviction in Israel's cause. This set of convictions left no room for psychic wounds in the national ethos, and impeded recognition of CSR for a quarter of a century after the founding of the state. It took another 25 years for an official declaration by Israel's legislature that battle shock is a war outcome and not a mental illness (see Chapter 1).

This same fear-justice loop also resonates with the conceptualizations of national resilience that have prevailed in Israel since the Al-Aqsa Intifada (2000–2004), and which enfold an implied linkage between patriotism and fear. These conceptualizations stem from the same old belief in the inuring power of love of one's homeland and, along with it, the desperate desire to believe in the absolute justice of Israel's goals and policies.[7]

Despite the great strides in recognizing war trauma as a legitimate injury, Israel still remains under the influence of the fear-justice loop. This loop underlies arguments that the recognition of war trauma has grown out of all proportion, that it encourages a "discourse of victimization,"[8] and even that it creates, among soldiers, a self-fulfilling prophecy of experiencing CSR or PTSD.[9] It likewise impedes the recognition of trauma suffered by IDF combatants due to harming or failing to prevent harm to Palestinian civilians.

Denial of war trauma is thus resurfacing, and is frequently accompanied by genuine resentment of the mirror that the traumatized soldiers hold up to society. This is particularly true for instances that extend the debate into addressing the overall Israeli policy in the Occupied Territories,[10] or the overall impact of the occupation on Israeli society.

The psychologically traumatized assess the world through heightened sensitivity for danger signs. They are hypersensitive to everyday sights, sounds, and events, and tend to be hostile and to erupt in angry outbursts. Their tense, volatile behavior goes hand in hand with a sense of helplessness and of psychic withdrawal. After all, trauma causes its casualties to relive the traumatizing event—endlessly, whether awake or asleep, in an obsessive fright of being caught in similar circumstances (Erikson 1995). At the same time, they are mired in a ceaseless effort to block reincursions of the terrifying event, and as a result avoid thoughts, feelings, and acts that might remind them of it. Such compulsive avoidance develops into emotional apathy that spreads to numerous areas of life and may manifest in indifference to the suffering of others, or withdrawal into a narrow psychological sphere restricted solely to oneself, or to her immediate social framework, in order to stave off further damage (Ayalon 1989).[11] In order to defend oneself from the distress that accompanies trauma, the psyche activates denial mechanisms that, while producing an illusion of adjustment, are also exhausting, particularly when hopes of change are repeatedly dashed (Breznitz 1983).

Israel's trauma ethos, like a societal PTSD, is shaping shared societal behaviors characterized by a combination of anxiety, aggressiveness, oversensitivity, apathy, and avoidance. This is a difficult claim to substantiate, given the difficulty of linking empirical data to the theoretical argument. However, as one distinguished psychologist, Rafael Moses, has noted, an analysis of Israel's behavioral traits as a state and as a society, whether directed inward or outward, demonstrates this clearly (Moses 1983). This claim also resonates with LaCapra's (2001) idea that trauma-related concepts are relevant to the analysis of sociopolitical processes no less than to processes of the individual. The following paragraphs explore several shared behaviors of Israeli society that reflect the trauma ethos.

Outwardly, these behaviors are manifest in hasty, sometimes disproportionate, reactions to criticism of Israel, which is immediately chalked up to anti-Semitism, and interpreting threats or specific provocations as existential dangers that elicit disproportionate responses that exacerbate existing security and political tensions. At the same time, foreigners' questions regarding life in the shadow of constant security threats typically trigger denial mechanisms (Breznitz 1983),[12] which represent a shared sense of detachment—a known defense mechanism in chronic trauma situations—as well as contradictory signs of coping. For example, studies of the mood of Israelis during the Al-Aqsa Intifada found an unusual combination of high levels of fear and helplessness, coupled with a strong sense of optimism (Zakai, quoted in Wiener 2004).[13] Although these findings may be indicative of resilience, it is undeniable that they also speak to activation of a self-illusion-of-adjustment defense mechanism. Both defense mechanisms—emotional detachment and self-illusion—are associated with adverse effects: the illusory adjustment reinforces tendencies to view war as destiny, reducing efforts to end the conflict, while the shared sense of detachment results in indifference to distress experienced by anyone whose social affiliation differs from one's own. This indifference is exhibited not only toward the suffering of those belonging to other nations—particularly the Palestinians—but also inwardly, toward large subsets of the domestic population. Worsening socioeconomic disparities are disregarded, as is the fate of the impoverished or disenfranchised sectors, especially those perceived as "other"—minorities, foreign workers, and refugees; indifference is growing toward spreading violence, unknown in Israel in the past.

Trauma researchers have repeatedly noted that a climate of trauma reenactment is a major cause of violence and that failure to deal with the plight of trauma victims can generate violence, not necessarily connected to the cause of trauma (Gobod-Madikizela 2008). This notion can be traced to an ideology of exaggerated entitlement and a sense that all is allowed in the name of self-defense (Volkan 2006),[14] to a predominant conviction of the necessity for self-preservation at the appearance of the smallest hint of threat, to inherited patterns of violence (McFarlane & Van der Kolk 1996), and to an overall atmosphere of restlessness. This conclusion aligns with findings of an international study that compared data from 80 countries and found a rise in the number of murders during postwar periods in all of those countries that had been involved in wars (Archer & Gartner, cited in Wiener 2004). The study found a direct correlation between a country's rising homicide rates and the number of its war casualties. In the authors' view, the findings point to a devaluing of human life and to a normalization of violence. Israel Police data also show that the incidence of civilian violence, including robbery and murder, has been steadily rising (Wiener 2004). While this trend can be traced to a myriad of causes, one cannot disregard the impact of Israel's trauma ethos, which legitimizes the use of force in the face of all perceived threats.

Throughout this book, I have shown that at two critical points in Israel's history, the Yom Kippur War (1973) and the Al-Aqsa Intifada (2000–2004), when society faced overwhelming dangers, the recognition of personal trauma began to take hold in spite of collective existential fears. Based on this country's underlying enslaving existential fears, these two points in time could have been expected to dampen recognition of war trauma, as these fears did in previous periods of severe threats, especially in the War of Independence. Paradoxically, however, CSR began to gain legitimacy in the wake of the Yom Kippur War (1973), and recognition of civilian acute stress reaction (ASR) increased during the Al-Aqsa Intifada.

The two events starkly differed: in contrast to the grave national danger that Israel faced in 1973 Yom Kippur War, the Al-Aqsa Intifada—although it occasioned great suffering and stress—did not represent an existential threat to the nation. The two crises, however, shared important similarities that facilitated the attitudinal change toward war trauma. The first was the increasing shift of attention to the suffering of the individual in war and terror, in addition to the collective national needs. Anger over the neglects of the Yom Kippur War and the changing of the guard between the combatants of 1948 and their children in 1973 made it emotionally possible for Israelis to admit to individual torments in war and their legitimacy, and to allow the idea of psychological trauma to pierce the heretofore-impenetrable armor of the indomitable-soldier myth. The Al-Aqsa Intifada expanded the space allotted to individual tolls of war to include civilians, whose suffering became conspicuous as the war infiltrated city and town centers. In some sense, Israelis had finally realized that the nation was made up of its individual members and not merely an essence on its own—an entity whose needs eclipsed its individual members.

The two events also shared an acceptance of security threats as a long-term reality with no end to war in sight. The reasons for the eradication of this hope were different in the two crises: the 1973 war smashed the Israeli illusion of power and proved that the sweeping victory of the Six-Day War failed to produce a new balance capable of preventing future wars; the Al-Aqsa Intifada demolished the belief in the possibility of peace. When the as-yet unimplemented peace agreements collapsed, and danger to the home front increased, Israelis lost hope in the likelihood of achieving peace. In both cases, the tendency to assume that the conflict was inevitable and irresolvable produced a new danger of its own: collective behavior and state policy that operated as a self-fulfilling prophecy.

The need to live with constant security threats since the birth of the country produced among Israelis a pattern of coping, made up of a camouflage of adjustment that disguises obsessive preoccupation with security. Psychiatrist Shlomo Breznitz, who conducted a study in confrontation-line towns in the 1980s, offers an illustration of such behavior. In answer to the question "What can you do with a shoe?"—a question designed to assess creative reasoning—one child responded, "Throw it at a terrorist" (Breznitz 1983).[15] Breznitz notes that this response highlights the gap between the outward display of apparently normal behavior and the inner psychic experience of constant preoccupation with menacing conditions. During the Al-Aqsa Intifada, a similarly superficial image of adjustment was reflected in a gap between the apparent return to everyday life and the profound effects of anxiety and tension on individuals. After each terrorist attack, life in Israel returned to normal—even in terms of restaurant patronage and bus travel—with astonishing rapidity, but each incident was also followed by a 35% increase in the number of fatal road accidents—a phenomenon that was traced directly to terrorism-induced stress among Israeli motorists (Stecklov & Goldstein 2004).[16]

In other words, despite the fact that a rapid resumption of normal activities is a desirable phenomenon that attests to high levels of resilience, it does not necessarily indicate recovery. It would not be an exaggeration to say that in Israel an image of recovery mainly reflects compliance with an overt societal demand to display such signs of resilience, while other, covert messages of permanent shared existential threats for the Jewish people are also being conveyed to civilians at the same time. These are the messages of the traumatic past. As happens in other large groups that suffered collective trauma in their past, collective memory—delivered by all memory agents—is of perpetual peril hovering over the nation (Volkan 2001). Rather than healing, such a social climate encourages superficial displays of adjustment at the expense of effortful work at genuine recovery. Novelist A. B. Yehoshua offered this apt description, after the terrorist attacks of 2004:

> You're mired in a sort of emotional helplessness and everything is completely arbitrary. Everything is incomprehensible. So we repress. So we sweep up the street right away. Clean up the blood. Get rid of the bus. And within an hour they're telling us on TV that life has returned to normal. Only the victims are being taken to Abu Kabir.[17]

Unhealed trauma, particularly when combined with persistent conflict, intensifies alienation and apathy, especially toward the designated enemy. In Israel's case, it blocks empathy toward the suffering of the civilian Palestinian population, which is seen as inextricably linked to the terrorist organizations. Research findings from the Al-Aqsa Intifada period indeed point to increasing public support for removing ethical limits of proportionality in military action, which have traditionally restricted the degree of force that the IDF exerts against the Palestinians.[18] In this context, it is worth noting that, while support for military activity is a logical and reasonable response during a wave of terrorism, reluctance to distinguish between civilians and terrorists indicates that that response has been shaped more by an ethos of trauma than by rational reasoning.

Reactivating the Trauma and Its Consequences

Such responses are not unique to Israel. Groups that have experienced national trauma transmit a shared mental representation of the trauma from generation to generation, which groups use as a prism to assess the present. Through this prism, contemporary threats are typically exaggerated and assume dimensions of immediate existential danger (Volkan 2006).[19] Under threat from an out-group, the present generation of traumatized individuals reactivates the past trauma in order to reinforce the group's shared identity and the conviction to combat the current threat (ibid.). However, since the trauma ethos impairs a true and practical evaluation of reality, such groups tend to choose violent responses, which eventually exacerbate the conflict instead of moderating it. This may be the background for what Daniel Bar-Tal calls "unifying the enemy," meaning a societal belief that even if the identity of the enemy changes, they are essentially the same (Bar-Tal 2007, pp. 118–119). These unconscious collective processes nurture Israelis' repetitive preoccupation with trauma, which turns the historical time of the Holocaust into a never-changing, everlasting epoch. Bar-Tal also suggests that the Israeli establishment deliberately reinforces this conceptual system and reworks the collective memory of the Holocaust into particularly potent symbols and metaphors, in an effort to strengthen national unity. The invocation of these code words awakens a sense of threat that triggers an entire cascade of emotions and behaviors, and reinforces both militancy and a perpetual climate of insecurity and threat.[20]

These unconscious processes call for yet another explanation. In a situation of protracted conflict, fear is undoubtedly a reasonable, even desirable response, but it normally subsides when the danger passes. A fear that, by contrast, arises out of a pathological pattern will persist despite changing conditions in a manner that is inconsistent with the world as it is. This is also true of human mourning. When mourning is "normal," the flood of emotions that it unleashes diminishes over time, while for traumatized people the memory of the event reactivates the feelings of fear, pain, and helplessness that they felt during the original incident in full force, time and time again (Foa et al. 2006).

Israelis are naturally ensnared by Holocaust memory both because there are still many living survivors and many more are second-generation survivors, and because it conforms to and even reinforces their trauma ethos. Israel's institutionalized commemoration of the Holocaust makes it impossible to process the trauma; rather, it reinforces what is effectively one more feature of post-traumatic disturbance: avoidance of anything related to the trauma. That is why the institutionalized commemoration of the Holocaust has no healing features. Instead, it strengthens the emotional-traumatic structure of Israeli society, which, for its part, remains inured to, and alienated from, the personal suffering of the Holocaust survivors themselves, and even neglects to care for weak and elderly survivors, as may be seen in the prevailing paucity of financial support for Holocaust survivors living under the poverty line.[21]

Avoidance, a known symptom of post-trauma, does not contradict the existing tendency toward obsessive preoccupation with the traumatic experience itself (see the introduction). On the contrary, obsessive engagement and avoidance reinforce each other. At the individual level, this mutual reinforcement is a major obstacle to recovery; at the collective level, it precludes any sense of relief or resolution of the shared traumatic experience. In this pattern of commemoration, society is controlled by the memory rather than controlling it, and is thereby deprived of the ability to distinguish between fear and distress caused by representations of the past and those rooted in current reality. This resonates with Pierre Nora's description of "moments of history torn away from the movement of history, then returned; no longer quite life, nor yet death, like shells on the shore when the sea of living memory has receded" (Nora 1989, p. 12).

Over the past decade, Israel has exhibited ever-stronger indications of psychological fatigue, manifested among other things in an increasing resignation with living in the shadow of war, which is seen as an inalterable situation, and in a major decline in public debate on potential resolutions of the conflict. In contrast to the agitated, vitriolic public debate that surrounded the Oslo Accords, in the period during and after the Al-Aqsa Intifada public attention focused on current reality rather than on efforts to change that reality. In the 1990s, despite the violent nature of the internal Israeli debate, which culminated in the assassination of Prime Minister Yitzhak Rabin, the social forces of that time believed that some kind of solution was on the horizon. Supporters of the peace process expected that the agreements would eventually be implemented and the terrorist attacks by Palestinian extremists who objected to the treaties would eventually cease; opponents of the process expected the agreements to be annulled and the previous state of affairs to be restored. In the 2000s, any orientation to the future was replaced by disappointment and despair of hope for change. The failure of the Camp David Summit and then prime minister Ehud Barak's declaration that Israel has no partner for peace[22] essentially redefined reality as a protracted military conflict unassailable by any possible military or political solution in the foreseeable future. This message, transmitted by the Israeli leadership without sparking any genuine public debate, channeled public attention through the limited prism of civilian psychological responses to life in terrorism's shadow.

Against this backdrop, the clinical discourse began to fulfill a social function that transcended the mental health sphere and enabled Israeli society to go on with life without viewing its situation as intolerable. This was not the first time that Israeli society assigned additional roles to mental health professionals, to provide support and solace through emotional and psychological guidance. As I have shown earlier in this book, Israel's war discourse had already been "hijacked" by the clinical discourse in the early 1990s. The political echelon's ineffectiveness during the Gulf War directed the helpless public to seek reassurance of experts, quoted enthusiastically and repeatedly by the media. This situation recurred during the Al-Aqsa Intifada, and again during the Second Lebanon War (2006), when the extreme unpreparedness of government social services once again left Israeli civilians leaderless in a traumatic reality. In their despair, the public turned to therapists and clinicians for comfort and fortification, who, in turn, took on an unintended role of filling the vacuum left by the leadership's silence. A similar pattern emerged in all three cases: therapists became the primary spokespersons in situations that were not primarily clinical, while the Israeli leadership fell silent and failed to offer any long-term vision or hope. This is an unfortunate situation. Although therapists' media-mediated messages effectively encourage the public in difficult times, these messages nevertheless mask the major issues raised by the war. From this perspective, the more efficient the clinical discourse proves to be in the short term, the more damaging it will be in the long term, inasmuch as it provides a convenient alternative, "releasing" the public from the inconvenient task of conducting meaningful discussions about ending the war. When unaccompanied by any meaningful political discourse oriented toward change, such a clinical discourse may engender a subtext of reconciliation with war's enduring nature—which, in a vicious circle, justifies the lack of any political discourse.

Efforts to resolve the conflict have indeed abated in recent years, and Israeli society, engrossed by its present wounds, is neglecting to consider the future and discuss peace initiatives thoroughly enough, finding it even more difficult to uproot its own discourse of victimization.

In his book about the survivors of Hiroshima, well-known trauma scholar Robert Jay Lifton discussed the importance of a sense of the self's symbolic wholeness, reflected in a feeling of coherence and meaning, to the recovery of trauma survivors, as well as the unconscious role of ideology and worldview in creating a bridge between self and world (Lifton 1991). In other words, trauma has a cultural and social content that also causes a major and profound identity crisis, and often shatters the basic paradigms through which people construct objective reality and link it to their subjective experiences in a meaningful and coherent way (Cohen & Farsha 2008).

This social and cultural content of trauma once again links the circles of individual and collective trauma—from stone to lake and back again—and urges us to examine yet another dimension of how Israel copes with its trauma ethos. From the 1980s on, Israel has been mired in an identity crisis that threatens the very core of its sense of self-image. The bitter dispute over the occupation and the means and goals of war has affected Israel's self-image; David has morphed into Goliath, not only in the eyes of the world but also in the eyes of a portion of its citizenry. Although some Israelis regard this new image as an excuse for their enemies' hatred and for the Jewish destiny of "dwelling apart," many others are unhappily persuaded by the new image of ferocious, uncaring might, and are gnawed by doubts as to the justice of their country's current cause. Neither group is free of the effects of trauma, and all Israelis are subject to the fear of an existential national catastrophe. Thus a new form of trauma emerged, in which the Israeli identity is itself split into victim and aggressor, with both sides beset by a sense of threat: in addition to the obvious sense of threat suffered by the victim of traumatic violence, the aggressor also feels threatened due to the collapse of their moral identity (Nadler & Shnabel 2008).

This split identity adds a new dimension to the familiar fear-justice loop, heightening its captive power. Emphasis on the victimization component of Israeli identity increases the threat to national resilience, reduces legitimization of war trauma, and reinforces processes that perpetuate the conflict. When the aggressor identity gains the upper hand, the threat to Israeli moral identity intensifies, the existence of psychological trauma that might call that identity into question is repressed, and the tendency to avoid self-examination or critical assessment of policies and behaviors pertaining to the conflict increases. When such criticism comes from the outside, Israel reacts forcefully and aggressively and interprets it as indications of old-new anti-Semitism. However, alongside the feverish and obsessive Israeli quest for manifestations of anti-Semitism, the country longs for other nations' recognition and friendship,[23] as was reflected in ordinary Israelis' passionate and enthusiastic response to President Barack Obama's speech in Jerusalem in March 2013. This convoluted and contradictory mode of behavior is reminiscent of the longing experienced by PTSD sufferers for a guiding hand at the same time they are secluding themselves and rejecting the outstretched hands of their families and loved ones.

The tortuous processes described earlier imprisons Israel within its traumatic experience and prevents it from considering its options rationally, free of past horrors. Awareness of the situation could potentially be a powerful healing force that might forge a new pathway out of the quagmire of fear, and save Israel from itself, perhaps even easing some of the country's persistent yearning for what we lost before it was born, and for what we hoped to be. Casualties of battle shock often wonder where the people they once were disappeared to. By extension, one can say that Israeli society is asking itself where the ethos of "who we once were," or who we wanted to be, has gone: a small, courageous nation fighting for its life in full confidence of the justice of its cause, and constantly striving for peace.

Notes

1. Over 22,000 fallen security-forces servicemen, 2,400 fallen civilians due to hostile acts, thousands of civilians wounded, and over 50,000 disabled IDF veterans with disability ratings exceeding 10%, at least 40% of whom were injured as a direct result of combat activity. Data analysis presented by Kuti Mor, director of the Defense Ministry's Disabled Rehabilitation Division, to the Public Committee to Assess Eligibility for Assistance from the Rehabilitation Divisions, 2010 (Goren Committee). This figure encompasses disabled IDF servicemen only and excludes those injured in road or other accidents unless they occurred during military exercises or operations. Six thousand soldiers and two thousand civilians are recognized as PTSD sufferers, but it is known that thousands of others have never been diagnosed despite the fact that they are afflicted with the syndrome at various levels of severity. The number of dead makes up 0.5% of the entire population, and the number of injured and families may be as high as 12%, not including Holocaust survivors and their families.
2. In 2008, there were a quarter of a million Holocaust survivors living in Israel (Brodsky et al. 2009).
3. See McEwan (1998, p. 140).
4. Collective trauma and national trauma are similar in meaning, and both terms are commonly used. Collective trauma can also take place in one of the communities of which a nation is composed, as when Hurricane Katrina struck New Orleans in 2005, killing 1,836 people and devastating the entire area.
5. Historian Dominick LaCapra regarded Freud's trauma-related concepts as relevant to and useful in the analysis of sociopolitical processes, no less than in the analysis of individual processes (Amos Goldberg's preface to LaCapra 2001).
6. On the presence of traumatic collective memory in Israeli life, see Shapira (1999); Segev (2000); Michman (1998); Don-Yehiya (1993).
7. See the section in Chapter 10 entitled "War Trauma and National Resilience."
8. NATAL Steering Committee, November 2009. Statement of Avi Bleich.
9. "If you don't suffer trauma you're not normal" (Levy interview, 2009).
10. The territories conquered by Israel in 1967, in the West Bank (also known as Judea and Samaria) and before 2005 also the Gaza Strip, from which Israel withdrew on that year.
11. Ayalon notes that activities aimed at increasing children's resilience in the face of security tension produce indifference to the suffering of others, since they emphasize processes of de-sensitization (Wiener 2004).
12. Similar denials were also expressed during the Al-Aqsa Intifada, despite contrary expressions of profound anxiety.
13. Alongside this optimism, 43% of Israelis reported a sense of helplessness, which, in half of the cases, had emerged since the Intifada.
14. Volkan's (2006) Chapter 10: the political ideology of entitlement and "chosen," "acute," and "hot" traumas (pp. 173–186).
15. Also see Breznitz's direct discussion of the inability of clinical diagnoses to encompass the effects of war on society.
16. The study isolated the impact of the terrorist attacks from other variables. My thanks to Dr. Yitzhak Levav for referring me to this article.
17. Quoted in Elran (2006, p. 31). The statement originally appeared in *Haaretz* on 19 March 2004. Abu Kabir is the Israeli forensic institute.
18. Ben-Dor et al. (2006) found that Jewish-Israeli militancy levels during the Second Intifada ranged from 4.19 to 4.64 on a scale of 1–6; Arian (2001) found a rise in support, from 31% in 1999 to 53% in 2001, for removing proportionality constraints upon the IDF.
19. See there also examples for transmission of chosen trauma in other places in the world. Volkan termed the phrase "chosen trauma" for this representation, as a signal to the unconscious's choice to add the representation of the trauma to the group's identity.
20. On this topic see also Nadler (1998).

21. This has become a major issue on the public agenda in recent years, which at the time of writing had yet to be satisfactorily resolved.
22. On prevailing opinions within the Israeli leadership regarding the chances for a successful peace process after the failure of the summer 2000 Camp David Summit, see Rabinovitch (2004).
23. See Israel's enthusiastic responses to Micronesia's support. One of many examples can be found on the Israeli government website, from the period of Ariel Sharon's premiership: www.pmo.gov.il/PMO/Archive/Events/2005/06/event220605.htm.

References

Arian, A. 2001, 'Israeli Public Opinion on National Security (Memorandum No. 60)', Jaffee Center for Strategic Studies, Tel Aviv University. Available from www.inss.org.il/upload/(FILE)1_190277683.pdf [29 May 2009].

Ayalon, A. 1989, 'The Psychological Price of the Security Situation', *H"T—Hovat Tze'aka!, Riv'on leHagut uleHinuch*, vol. 2, pp. 32–40. (Hebrew)

Bar-Tal, D. 2007, *Living with the Conflict: Socio-Psychological Analysis of Jewish Society in Israel*, Carmel, Jerusalem.

Ben-Dor, G., Canetti, D., & Halperin, E. 2006, 'The Social Component of National Resilience', presentation given at Sixth Herzliya Conference, Herzliya. Available from www.herzliyaconference.org/_Uploads/2131hosen_heb.pdf [30 January 2010]. (Hebrew)

Bilu, Y., & Witztum, E. 2000, 'War-Related Loss and Suffering in Israeli Society: an Historical Perspective', *Israel Studies*, vol. 5, no. 2, p. 1.

Bodnar, J. 1998, 'Review of Arthur G. Neal, *National Trauma and Collective Memory: Major Events in the American Century*', *H-Pol, H-Net Reviews*. Available from www.h-net.org/reviews/showrev.php?id-2260.

Breznitz, S. 1983, 'The Noble Challenge of Stress', in *Stress in Israel*, ed. S. Breznitz, Van Nostrand Reinhold, New York, pp. 265–274.

Brodsky, J., Sharon, A., King, Y., Be'er, S., & Shnoor, Y. 2009, 'Holocaust Survivors in Israel: Population Estimates, Demographic, Health and Social Characteristics, and Needs'. Available from http://brookdaleheb.jdc.org.il/?CategoryID=156&ArticleID=70 [21 May 2010]. (Hebrew; English at: http://brookdale.jdc.org.il/_Uploads/PublicationsFiles/553-10-Holocaust-Survivors-ES-ENG.pdf)

Cohen, M., & Farsha, E. 2008, 'Social and Cultural Contexts of Combat Stress Reaction: War Trauma as Identity Crisis', *Hebrew Psychology* [electronic version]. Available from www.hebpsy.net/articles.asp?id-1781 [27 July 2010]. (Hebrew)

Don-Yehiya, E. 1993, 'Memory and Political Culture: Israeli Society and the Holocaust', *Studies in Contemporary Jewry*, vol. 9, pp. 139–162.

Eliot, M., Bishop, K., & Stokes, P. 2004, 'Societal PTSD? Historic Shock in Northern Ireland', *Psychotherapy and Politics International*, vol. 2, no. 1, pp. 1–16.

Elran, M. 2006, 'Israel's National Resilience: the Influence of the Second Intifada on Israeli Society', Jaffee Center for Strategic Studies at Tel Aviv University, Memorandum no. 81, pp. 5–6. (Hebrew)

Erikson, K. T. 1978, *Everything in Its Path: Destruction of Community in the Buffalo Creek Flood*, Simon & Schuster, New York.

Erikson, K. T. 1995, 'Notes on Trauma and Community' in *Trauma: Explorations in Memory*, ed. C. Caruth, Johns Hopkins University Press, Baltimore, pp. 183–199.

Foa, E., Doron, M., & Yadin, E. 2006, *Prolonged Exposure: Guide to Treatment of Post-Traumatic Stress Disorder*, Community Stress Prevention Center, Kiryat Shmona.

Gobod-Madikizela, P. 2008, 'Transforming Trauma in the Aftermath of Gross Human Rights Abuses: Making Public Spaces Intimate through the South African Truth and Reconciliation Commission' in *The Social Psychology of Intergroup Reconciliation*, eds. A. Nadler, T. A. Malloy, & D. J. Fisher, Oxford University Press, New York, pp. 57–73.

LaCapra, D. 2001, *Writing History, Writing Trauma*, Johns Hopkins University Press, Baltimore.

Lifton, R. J. 1991, *Death in Life: Survivors of Hiroshima*, University of North Carolina Press, Chapel Hill.

McEwan, I. 1998, *Black Dogs*, Anchor Books, New York.

McFarlane, A. C., & Van der Kolk, B. A. 1996, 'Trauma and Its Challenge to Society' in *Traumatic Stress: the Effect of Overwhelming Experience on Mind, Body and Society*, eds. A. C. McFarlane & B. A. Van Der Kolk, Guildford, New York, pp. 25–45.

Michman, D. 1998, *Holocaust and Holocaust Research*, Moreshet, Tel Aviv. (Hebrew)

Moses, R. 1983, 'Emotional Response to Stress in Israel: a Psychoanalytic Perspective' in *Stress in Israel*, ed. S. Breznits, Van Nostrand Reinhold, New York, pp. 114–137.

Nadler, A. 1998, 'Incitement and Political Murder' in *Political Assassination: the Murder of Rabin and Political Assassinations in the Middle East*, ed. C. Y. Liebman, Yitzhak Rabin Center for Israel Studies and Am Oved, Tel Aviv. (Hebrew)

Nadler, A., & Shnabel, N. 2008, 'Instrumental and Socio-Emotional Paths to Intergroup Reconciliation and the Needs-Based Model of Socio-Emotional Reconciliation' in *The Social Psychology of Intergroup Reconciliation*, eds. A. Nadler, T. A. Malloy, & D. J. Fisher, Oxford University Press, New York, pp. 37–56.

Neal, A. G. 1998, *National Trauma and Collective Memory: Major Events in the American Century*, M. E. Sharpe, Armonk, NY.

Nora, P. 1989, 'Between Memory and History: Les Lieux de Memoire', *Representations*, vol. 26, special issue, *Memory and Counter-Memory*, pp. 7–24.

Rabinovitch, I. 2004, *Waging Peace: Israel and the Arabs, 1948–2003*, Princeton University Press, Princeton.

Segev, T. 2000, *The Seventh Million: the Israelis and the Holocaust*, Macmillan, New York.

Shapira, A. 1999, *Land and Power: the Zionist Resort to Force, 1881–1948*, Stanford University Press, Stanford.

Shay, J. 2010, *Achilles in Vietnam: Combat Trauma and the Undoing of Character*, Simon and Schuster, New York.

Solomon, Z., Weissman, M, Levi, G., Fried, B., Mikolinsar, M., Benbenishty, R., Florian, V., & Bleich, A. 1992, 'From Front Line to Home Front: a Study of Secondary Traumatization', *Family Process*, vol. 31, no. 3, pp. 289–302.

Stecklov, G., & Goldstein, J. R. 2004, 'Terror Attacks Influence Driving Behavior in Israel', *Proceedings of the National Academy of Sciences* (USA), vol. 101, no. 40, pp. 14551–14556.

Volkan, V. 2006, *Killing in the Name of Identity: a Study of Bloody Conflicts*, Pitchstone, Charlottesville.

Volkan, V. D. 2001, 'Transgenerational Transmissions and Chosen Traumas: an Aspect of Large-Group Identity', *Group Analysis*, vol. 34, no. 1, pp. 79–97.

Wiener, Z. 2004, 'Individual and Societal Reactions to Ongoing Terror in Israel', *Journal of Ambulatory Care Management*, vol. 28, no. 1, pp. 80–85.

Epilogue

When I completed my work on this book, I tried to elucidate, for myself, the feeling that filled me the moment the keyboard finally was silent—a feeling that I would like my readers to share in their own hearts. It is difficult to deconstruct emotions and put them in words, but perhaps the most important thing for me is to underscore the powerful impact of collective memory and trauma ethos. These two burdens of history ensnare us in vicious circles of unending wars, while at the same time preventing us from taking full responsibility for all forms of war victims, and hindering our empathy for the trauma of other groups. This is true of all wars and all peoples, and it is especially true for Israel.

The dream of a Jewish state was built on an amalgam of exigency and fear, national aspirations, hope for a better future, and even visions of reestablishing ancient traditions of life in the Holy Land. Alongside the element of necessity driven by oppression, threatened annihilation, and the eternal Jewish destiny of exile and anti-Semitism, sublime dreams also emerged—longing for a Hebrew culture and a humanistic society, and a desire for national existence in the spirit of the revolutions of 1848—the "Springtime of the Peoples."

When the Jewish people began to follow the Zionist dreamers into the "Land of Yisrael,"[1] the land became populated not only with people but also with infinite memories. Women and men arrived with bundles of memories on their backs and suitcases of hope in their hands. These were memories of childhood homes and distant landscapes —landscapes that had been abandoned by young people seeking to escape a world of humiliation, hatred, and injustice, of teeming, suffocating ghettos where there was no room to spread one's wings and soar to heights of cultural or social creativity. These were memories of atrocity, horror, forced flight, and annihilation. From the west and from the east, from the north and from the south they came. Memory crowded upon memory, filling the air like a thick vapor, crowding out the fragile seeds of longing for a better life—a life founded on liberty and justice, a culture of freedom and solidarity, and care for the weak.

I have always been aware of the power of traumatic memories, especially for a nation whose history is steeped in horror and that experienced a collective trauma of such immense proportions as the Holocaust. But the story of how Israel has coped with war trauma brought home to me even more strongly the connection between the individual and collective, and the destructive power of memories that are transmitted from generation to generation unprocessed, inhibiting healing. I would like to raise awareness of this dragon of memory, for only when we dare to look head-on at the abyss of horror within us will we be able to tame the beast, rather than being controlled by it. I believe that understanding Israel's dialogue with war trauma is a step in this direction, and a way out of the trap of memory that is already overflowing, overwhelming us, and stifling our ability to think differently.

A moment before typing the book's final sentence, I realized that the end of this book marks the beginning of a new journey for me, a quest for the means of converting the negative effects of personal and collective traumatic memory into positive forces of empathy, openness, and mutual understanding. I hope that this is no naïve fantasy. Despite the menacing and perpetual power of memory, new voices have emerged in recent years to argue that collective memory and traumatic experiences can be mobilized differently, in the service of reconciliation, and employed as an impetus for attitudinal change—facilitating recognition of the shared suffering that war causes to all parties affected by it (Keynan 2009).

This will be a long journey, riddled with obstacles, but it holds great promise. First and foremost for the war-trauma casualties themselves: liberation from the collective ethos of trauma will make it easier for us to acknowledge their pain and to recognize our responsibility to them and for their fate. But this journey embodies an even more daring hope, for Israeli society as a whole—to come to terms with its power to shape its own future; to forge a path out of horror to a place where one still has a chance of seeing the dawn "sparkle in its freshness like an open gate."[2]

Notes

1. The Land of Israel (Eretz Yisrael) is the Hebrew name for the territory that God promised to Abraham. In other languages, this is also called the Promised Land, the Holy Land, or the Land of Milk and Honey. The Jews used the name Eretz Yisrael for the area that was subject to the British Mandate (1922–1948) until Israel's independence.
2. L. Goldberg, 1986, "End of Summer Songs, I. The Domain", *Poems*, part 3, Sifriat Poalim, Bnei-Brak, p. 244 (Hebrew).

Reference

Keynan, I. 2009, 'Collective Memory and Intergroup Leadership: Israel as a Case Study', in *Crossing the Divide: Intergroup Leadership in a World of Difference*, ed. T. L. Pittinsky, Harvard Business Press, Boston, pp. 219–230.

Index

For Product Safety Concerns and Information please contact our EU representative GPSR@taylorandfrancis.com
Taylor & Francis Verlag GmbH, Kaufingerstraße 24, 80331 München, Germany

www.ingramcontent.com/pod-product-compliance
Ingram Content Group UK Ltd.
Pitfield, Milton Keynes, MK11 3LW, UK
UKHW011013180926
475701UK00004B/717